QUICK & EASY LOW-FODMAP DIET COOKBOOK

Discover an Endless Array of Flavorful Recipes to Support IBS Symptoms, Boost Digestive Health, and Bring Comfort to Your Meals 60-Day Meal Plan Included

Elodie Vance

QUICK & EASY LOW-FODMAP DIET COOKBOOK

TABLE OF CONTENTS

CHAPTER 10: DESSERT DELIGHTS 76

CHAPTER 11: BOOSTING FLAVORS 85

CHAPTER 12: CONCLUSION AND FINAL THOUGHTS 94

CHAPTER 13: IN-DEPTH 60-DAY MEAL PLAN 100

CHAPTER 1: INTRODUCTION AND WELCOME

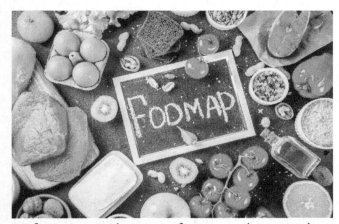

Welcome to a journey that promises not just relief but a revival of the joy in eating. If you're navigating through the choppy waters of digestive issues like IBS, you've probably faced days when your stomach seemed like an enigma, reacting unpredictably to foods that others can enjoy freely. It's frustrating, isn't it? Overcoming this challenge is what brings us together in these pages.

Imagine stepping into a world where your dietary choices empower you, rather than restrict you. That's the essence of the LOW-FODMAP diet, and this cookbook is your map to mastering it. Here, you'll find not just recipes, but companionship and a guide that appreciates the complexity of your needs.

Why LOW-FODMAP, you might ask? The science is compelling. This diet has been clinically acknowledged for its ability to alleviate and manage the symptoms of digestive distress caused by foods high in certain carbohydrates that are challenging to digest. But, sticking to such a diet can be daunting. The thought of navigating grocery store aisles or cooking daily meals can seem overwhelming. I understand that feeling all too well, which is why this book is designed to simplify, not complicate.

Through this cookbook, I aim to reintroduce you to the pleasure of cooking and eating every meal with confidence. Gone are the days when managing your symptoms meant settling for bland, uninspiring dishes.

Together, we'll unlock a spectrum of flavors that keep your meals exciting and your belly calm. From hearty breakfasts to satisfy your morning appetite, to fulfilling dinners that can please even those without dietary restrictions we've got a plate for every taste.

Not just meals, but this guide is about celebration of food, of wellbeing, and of the peace that comes with understanding what works for your body. Let's embark on this culinary adventure together, with each recipe not just feeding your body, but also nourishing your soul and bringing back the joy in your dining experiences. Welcome to my kitchen let the cooking begin!

1.1 GRASPING THE LOW-FODMAP DIET

Imagine walking through a maze; each turn represents a choice of foods that could either trigger discomfort or provide relief. This is often the daily reality for those with sensitive digestive systems. The LOW-FODMAP diet is much like a map through that maze, providing clear guidelines and choices that help reduce gastrointestinal symptoms for many. So, let's explore this approach, understanding its fundamentals, and how it promises a better quality of life.

The term "FODMAP" stands for Fermentable Oligo-, Di-, Mono-saccharides And Polyols. These are short-chain carbohydrates and sugar alcohols found in various foods, which, in sensitive individuals, are not efficiently absorbed by the small intestine. When these unabsorbed sugars reach the colon, they ferment, causing the all-too-familiar symptoms of IBS, such as bloating, gas, abdominal pain, constipation, and diarrhea.

Introduced by researchers at Monash University in Australia, the LOW-FODMAP diet has become a beacon of hope for millions. This diet isn't about wholesale dietary restrictions but focuses on limiting foods high in these fermentable sugars, thereby managing the volume of fermentable substrates available to intestinal bacteria.

The Phases of the LOW-FODMAP Diet:
Starting on this diet is more than just a series of food swaps. It typically unfolds in three strategic phases:

1. **Elimination:** This initial phase involves removing high-FODMAP foods from one's diet for a period, usually 4-6 weeks. This is the time to observe how your body responds in the absence of these triggers.

2. **Reintroduction:** Gradually reintroducing foods helps to pinpoint specific triggers and understand how much of a high-FODMAP food can be tolerated. It's a delicate balance, aiming not to overwhelm the gut while gauging its response.

3. **Personalization:** The final phase is about creating a long-term eating plan based on the learnings from the reintroduction phase. This personalized plan allows flexibility and ensures a nutritionally balanced diet while keeping symptoms at bay.

Navigating the LOW-FODMAP Diet:
It's crucial to understand that this diet isn't about deprivation but about discovery and adaptation. You start by stripping the diet back to basics and then reintroduce foods methodically to decode your body's responses. In practice, the diet dictates avoiding items like onions, garlic, certain fruits such as apples and mangoes, dairy products high in lactose, wheat-based products, and artificial sweeteners like sorbitol and mannitol, among others. Instead, you can enjoy foods like carrots, cucumbers, grapes, strawberries, lactose-free dairy, quinoa, and tofu, to name a few.

The Challenges and Triumphs:
Navigating this diet, especially in the early days, can be daunting. The fear of accidentally consuming a high-FODMAP food and triggering symptoms is common. Moreover, due to the restrictive phase of the diet, there's a potential risk of inadequate nutrient intake if not properly managed. Therefore, education, careful meal planning, and sometimes the guidance of a nutritionist are paramount.

Despite these challenges, the successes of the LOW-FODMAP diet weave stories of regained control and revived spirits. It's not merely about managing a condition but about reclaiming the joy that comes from a diverse and delicious diet.

A Lifelong Commitment?
As we delve deeper into the nuances of managing digestive health through diet, it becomes evident that the LOW-FODMAP approach isn't typically a lifelong diet. Instead, it's a tool to gain insights into what your body can tolerate and how you can adjust your eating habits to live comfortably and without fear.

In this context, the diet is both a diagnostic tool and a lifestyle guide. It offers a structured way to identify foods that trigger symptoms, teaches moderation, and helps create a balanced diet that celebrates a wide array of food options.

As we journey through this cookbook, remember that each recipe is designed not just to adhere to the LOW-FODMAP guidelines but to ensure that every meal is a step toward symptom relief and culinary delight. The path may seem complex at first glance, but it leads to a more insightful relationship with your food and your body. Here, the focus isn't only on the foods you can't eat, but more importantly, on the delicious meals you *can* eat.

1.2 ADVANTAGES AND CHALLENGES OF THIS DIET

Embarking on the LOW-FODMAP diet often feels like setting out on a journey where the landscape shifts between exhilarating exploration and challenging terrain. It offers significant benefits, certainly, but it's also fraught with its own unique set of hurdles. Herein lies an opportunity to understand the dual nature of this diet its perks and pitfalls to help you traverse this path with informed intentions.

The Advantages of the LOW-FODMAP Diet

Perhaps the most profound benefit of the LOW-FODMAP diet is the relief it offers from the troubling and often debilitating symptoms of gastrointestinal disorders such as irritable bowel syndrome (IBS). The reduction in symptoms can significantly enhance quality of life, making daily activities more enjoyable and less fraught with anxiety around potential digestive discomfort.

1. **Symptom Relief:** Many who adopt this diet experience a considerable decrease in the frequency and intensity of symptoms such as bloating, gas, diarrhea, and constipation. This relief often begins within just a few weeks of starting the elimination phase.

2. **Improved Diagnostics:** By systematically eliminating and reintroducing foods, you gain a clearer understanding of which foods trigger your symptoms. This insight allows for a more tailored diet that can strategically exclude only those foods that cause discomfort, rather than broadly restricting diet.

3. **Nutritional Awareness:** Following this diet requires you to become acutely aware of what you're eating. This heightened awareness often improves overall dietary habits, as it encourages the consumption of a variety of whole foods and home-prepared meals.

4. **Empowerment and Control:** Understanding which foods you can eat without symptoms can empower you to make choices that prevent discomfort. This sense of control can lead to increased confidence and decreased anxiety related to eating.

Addressing the Challenges

Despite its many benefits, the LOW-FODMAP diet is not without its challenges. It requires significant changes to your eating habits and lifestyle, which can be demanding.

1. **Complexity and Restrictiveness:** Initially, the diet can appear overwhelming due to the strict limitations on certain common foods known to be high in FODMAPs, such as onions, garlic, wheat, and some fruits. Learning to navigate these restrictions can be a daunting task.

2. **Social and Emotional Impact:** Dietary restrictions can affect social interactions and enjoyment associated with dining out or sharing meals with others. It can feel isolating to have a plate full of 'can't haves' during social gatherings.

3. **Risk of Nutritional Deficiencies:** If not carefully managed, the diet can lead to deficiencies in certain nutrients. This is particularly true during the elimination phase, where multiple food groups might be significantly limited or entirely avoided.

4. **Time and Effort for Meal Planning:** The need to read labels closely, plan meals meticulously, and perhaps cook separate dishes can add extra layers of effort and time commitment to daily routines.

Navigating Through the Challenges

The successful adoption of the LOW-FODMAP diet involves striking a balance between the benefits and the challenges. Here are a few strategies to mitigate the difficulties:

- **Educate Yourself and Others:** Understanding the scientific basis and the practical implementations of the diet can alleviate much of the anxiety surrounding it. Educating friends and family can also make social meals less stressful.
- **Seek Professional Guidance:** Consulting dietitians who specialize in the LOW-FODMAP diet can provide personalized advice and reassurance, helping to ensure that your diet remains balanced and beneficial.
- **Use Technology:** Various apps and resources are designed to help manage the LOW-FODMAP diet, offering meal ideas, tracking symptoms, and even scanning product barcodes to check for FODMAPs.
- **Plan Ahead:** Meal prepping and planning can mitigate much of the stress associated with adhering to a restrictive diet, especially when busy or dining out.

The Path Forward

Transitioning to a LOW-FODMAP lifestyle can be likened to learning a new language. It might be cumbersome at first, but with practice, it becomes a fluent part of your life, unlocking new joys in eating and wellbeing.

Embrace the process as a journey of discovery about your body and its needs, which can lead to a more mindful and healthful way of living. While challenges exist, the strategies to navigate them are effective and can lead to sustained success. Remember, the ultimate goal is not just to follow a diet but to enjoy a richer, more active life, free from the burden of digestive discomfort.

1.3 HOW THIS COOKBOOK WILL ASSIST YOU

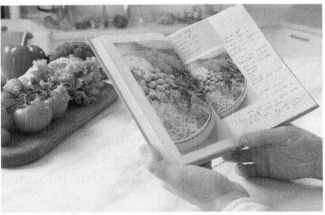

Embarking on the LOW-FODMAP journey introduces a new chapter in your culinary life a chapter filled with understanding, control, and relief. This cookbook, crafted with both care and expertise, is designed to be a companion that walks alongside you as you navigate your dietary needs. It bridges the gap between medical advice and everyday living, offering practical solutions for a smoother transition into a LOW-FODMAP lifestyle.

At its core, this cookbook aims to demystify the complexities of the LOW-FODMAP diet, making it accessible and manageable. It is structured to ease you into the diet gradually, ensuring you understand the why and how before jumping into the what. This approach is essential, as it fosters a deeper understanding and a more sustainable adoption of the diet.

Guided Support Through Each Phase

Educational Foundation: Before you dive into cooking, the cookbook lays a solid educational foundation about FODMAPs what they are, why they can cause distress, and how manipulating their intake can alleviate this distress. This knowledge is pivotal, as it empowers you to make informed decisions beyond the scope of this cookbook.

Phase-by-Phase Guidance: Reflecting the three phases of the LOW-FODMAP diet, the cookbook is segmented into clear, manageable parts. Each section supports one of the diet's phases from elimination to reintroduction and personalization. Such structured guidance helps prevent the feeling of being overwhelmed and ensures that each step is a building block to the next.

Tailoring to Taste and Tolerance: As you explore which FODMAPs you can tolerate and in what quantities, this cookbook serves as a guide to tweaking recipes to meet your personal tolerance levels. This individualized approach not only helps in managing symptoms but also in expanding your diet with confidence.

Overcoming the Challenges with Practical Tools

Simplifying Complex Diets: The fear of starting a restrictive diet often lies in its perceived complexity. This cookbook simplifies the process with clear, easy-to-follow recipes and tips for modifying them according to your specific needs. Whether it's substituting an ingredient or adjusting portion sizes, you'll find guidance that respects your body's limits without compromising on flavor.

Time-Saving Techniques: Understanding the time constraints and the effort involved in preparing special meals, especially when you're managing other aspects of life, the cookbook offers quick, practical meal ideas. These include timesaving tips for meal preparation and suggestions for effectively using leftovers, making it easier to adhere to the diet without feeling burdened.

Emotional and Social Support: A significant aspect of dietary management is dealing with the emotional and social implications. This cookbook acknowledges these challenges and provides advice on how to handle social situations, from explaining your dietary needs with confidence to hosting gatherings where everyone enjoys the food without singling out the dietary restrictions.

Nourishing Body and Soul

Holistic Nutrition: Beyond managing symptoms, this cookbook focuses on overall health and well-being. It ensures that the recipes are balanced, nutritious, and conducive to a healthy lifestyle. Aspect of culinary pleasure is overlooked. Recipes are designed to delight the taste buds, ensuring that meals are enjoyed and not just tolerated.

Inspiring Creativity in the Kitchen: With an array of recipes from basic staples to exotic dishes, the cookbook encourages you to expand your culinary skills. The exploration of international cuisines not only adds variety but also introduces new flavors and techniques, keeping the excitement alive in your cooking journey.

Fostering Independence: Ultimately, the goal of this cookbook is to equip you with the skills and confidence to create your own LOW-FODMAP recipes. By understanding the fundamentals of what makes a dish LOW-FODMAP, you'll be able to adapt almost any recipe, granting you greater flexibility and independence in your diet.

A Journey Shared

This cookbook doesn't just provide you with recipes; it accompanies you on a journey towards better health and greater happiness. It's a testament to the fact that dietary restrictions don't have to mean culinary restrictions. With each page, you'll find yourself more empowered, more knowledgeable, and more in control of your digestive health. This book is here to show that with the right ingredients, a pinch of creativity, and a dash of knowledge, your meals can transform from mundane to extraordinary, all while keeping your stomach soothed and your spirits high.

In essence, *Quick & Easy Low-FODMAP Diet Cookbook* isn't just about eating; it's about living well, with every meal a celebration of life beyond digestive distress. Welcome to a new way of eating, where your diet is not a limitation but an exploration of tastes, textures, and the joys of finding what works best for your body.

CHAPTER 2: DIET ESSENTIALS OVERVIEW

Welcome to the core of your low-FODMAP journey, where familiarizing yourself with the essentials of the diet isn't just important it's transformative. Understanding the nature of FODMAPs and recognizing which foods to embrace or avoid is your first, crucial step toward a happier, healthier gut.

Imagine standing in your kitchen, the heart of your home, surrounded by foods that once triggered discomfort and confusion. Now, see it transformed into a sanctuary where every shelf and every pantry holds promise, not peril. This is what understanding the fundamentals of the low-FODMAP diet can offer you. FODMAPs, which stand for Fermentable Oligosaccharides, Disaccharides, Monosaccharides, and Polyols, are carbohydrates that can cause irritation in the gut of some people, leading to symptoms that can disrupt your day-to-day life.

Here in this chapter, we begin by laying down a clear, nurturing path through these complex names and processes. It's important to recognize the dual face of FODMAPs while they are present in a wide array of nutritious foods, their fermentation process can create chaos in sensitive digestive systems. By distinguishing between high and low FODMAP foods, you equip yourself with the knowledge to make choices that align with your body's needs.

Remember when meal planning felt like navigating a minefield? We'll shift from that uncertainty to empowerment, as you learn not just to identify these foods, but to understand why certain ones can be a green light for your gut, while others are a stop sign. This chapter takes you by the hand and gently guides you through recognizing these foods in the grocery aisles, understanding food labels, and adapting your favorite dishes with low-FODMAP alternatives that don't cut corners on flavor.

Each element of this diet can be tailored to fit your unique lifestyle and dietary needs, transforming the daunting into the doable. Through this insightful exploration, prepare to reclaim your kitchen, enjoy your meals, and revitalize your health with every bite you take.

2.1 UNDERSTANDING FODMAPs

Delving into the intricacies of FODMAPs reveals a tale woven not only through the foods we eat but how our bodies interact with these seemingly innocuous ingredients. As you embark on this educational journey, it's like peeling back layers of an everyday mystery, revealing how certain carbohydrates are playing a game of disguise and surprise with your digestive system.

The acronym FODMAP stands for Fermentable Oligosaccharides, Disaccharides, Monosaccharides, and Polyols. These categories encompass a variety of sugars and fibers that some individuals find difficult to digest. What makes FODMAPs particularly intriguing and sometimes troubling is their fermentable nature, which causes them to be metabolized by the bacteria in our gut. This fermentation process can lead to increased water and gas in the intestines, which for many, results in discomfort, bloating, and other more severe symptoms associated with conditions like Irritable Bowel Syndrome (IBS).

To truly understand FODMAPs, one must look beyond the complexities of their names:

- **Oligosaccharides:** Found in foods like wheat, onions, and garlic, oligosaccharides are carbohydrates composed of simple sugars linked in chains. They elude digestion in the upper gut and ferment in the lower colon, leading to gas and bloating.

- **Disaccharides:** Lactose is the poster child here, prevalent in dairy products such as milk and soft cheeses. For those with lactose intolerance, the disaccharide can't be broken down efficiently, resulting in gastrointestinal distress upon consumption.
- **Monosaccharides:** Fructose, when present in greater quantities than glucose, can be troublesome. High-fructose foods like apples, honey, and high-fructose corn syrup can draw water into the intestine, causing an upset.
- **Polyols:** These sugar alcohols such as sorbitol and mannitol are found in some fruits and vegetables and used as artificial sweeteners. They can pull water into the bowel and ferment, causing symptoms.

Understanding these categories helps demystify why certain healthful foods can still lead to unpleasant reactions in some people. It's akin to finding out that a trusted friend has unwittingly been causing you distress. With knowledge comes power, the power to adapt and choose nourishment that heals rather than harms.

The challenge with managing a low-FODMAP diet lies not just in identifying these compounds but in recognizing their quantities in food, as many healthy foods contain FODMAPs but can be tolerated in small amounts. Thus, portion control and moderation play crucial roles. The relationship between FODMAPs and the gut environment is a dynamic interplay; not everyone will respond the same way to the same food. This is where the personalization of the diet becomes key, a testament to the intricate and unique nature of each individual's digestive system.

The laboratory of life presents itself in your kitchen every day. As you experiment with reducing and moderating these FODMAPs, you'll likely notice a pattern of symptoms that correspond with specific foods. It's a form of detective work, where your payoff isn't just solving a case but achieving a happier, less disruptive life. This actionable intelligence empowers you to make informed decisions about your diet.

Consider the story of Julia, a vibrant teacher who loved her job but dreaded her daily battle with bloating and fatigue. It wasn't until she understood the impact of high-FODMAP foods on her body that she was able to replace onions, garlic, and wheat in her meals with low-FODMAP alternatives like green onions, garlic-infused oils, and spelt bread. Julia's energy returned, her discomfort waned, and she felt in control again.

Your journey with FODMAPs might also be revealing. Start with an elimination phase, designed to clear your system of all high-FODMAP foods. Then, carefully reintroduce them one by one, gauging your body's reactions to find your personal thresholds. This tailored approach helps you cultivate a diet that respects your body's limits while ensuring nutritional balance.

In essence, understanding FODMAPs isn't merely academic it's a key to unlocking better health and greater enjoyment of life's pleasures, including the joy of good food. So, as you embark on this exploration, remember that each meal, each choice, is a step toward a more understanding and harmonious relationship with your body. This is not just about avoiding certain foods; it's about embracing an informed way of eating that promotes a robust, vibrant life. Your guidebook through this journey is your awareness and the insights from each meal that contribute to a holistic understanding of how food affects you personally.

2.2 RECOGNIZING HIGH AND LOW FODMAP FOODS

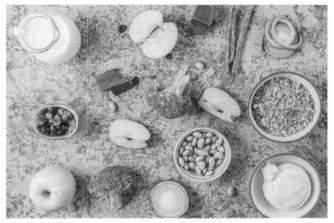

Embarking on the low-FODMAP journey, the art of distinguishing between high and low FODMAP foods becomes a pivotal skill. This knowledge acts like a compass, guiding you through the grocery aisles and menu selections with confidence and ease. For anyone grappling with digestive sensitivities, mastering this skill is akin to learning a new language the language of your own body's responses to food.

Each person's relationship with food is as unique as their fingerprint, and understanding which foods harbor high amounts of FODMAPs and which do not could be likened to navigating one's way through a detailed map of dietary choices. This map leads you through rough terrains (high FODMAP zones) and safe havens (low FODMAP areas), enabling you to make informed, beneficial choices.

High FODMAP foods are like the hidden rocks in an otherwise serene landscape, causing turmoil for those with a sensitive digestive system. These foods include certain fruits like apples, pears, and mangoes, which contain excess fructose. Vegetables such as onions and garlic are major contributors of fructans, while dairy products rich in lactose like milk and soft cheeses, and grains such as wheat and rye, also sit prominently on the high FODMAP list. Furthermore, sweeteners such as honey and products containing high fructose corn syrup or sugar alcohols like sorbitol and mannitol can also trigger symptoms.

Transitioning to the low FODMAP sanctuaries brings relief and variety. Embellish your plate with bananas, oranges, and grapes, which are kinder to your guts. Vegetables such as carrots, bell peppers, and cucumbers along with leafy greens like spinach and kale nourish without distress. For dairy lovers, lactose-free options and hard cheeses offer creamy delight without discomfort. Quinoa, rice, and oats stand as hearty, soothing grain choices. In the realm of sweeteners, choices shift towards maple syrup and table sugar, which are typically tolerated better.

Experiencing the journey from a high to a low FODMAP diet could be thought of as a trek from a tumultuous sea into calming waters. Take Sarah, a university student who loved experiencing the eclectic mix of the campus dining hall but often found herself battling severe abdominal pains afterward. It wasn't until she consulted with a dietitian and discovered the impact of high FODMAP foods that she started to map out her meals differently. Learning to choose sushi rolls made with rice (a low FODMAP food) instead of ones with onion-filled sauces transformed her dining experience from painful to pleasurable.

Recognizing these foods does require attentiveness and diligence. It's not just about reading labels for hidden ingredients but also managing portion sizes as even low FODMAP foods can escalate into high FODMAP territories if consumed in large amounts. This nuanced understanding adds layers to your meal planning incorporating not just what to eat, but how much and when.

Grocery shopping transforms from a chore to an investigative mission. Armed with the knowledge of high and low FODMAP foods, you can navigate labels and ingredient lists with the precision of a detective. It's an empowering process, one that slowly replaces uncertainty with confidence.

Eating out, once a field ripe with potential landmines, becomes less daunting. By understanding menu items and their likely FODMAP content, choosing wisely becomes second nature. Questions for your server become more pointed and informed, ensuring that eating out remains a joy, not a gamble.

For those beginning this journey, the transition may seem overwhelming at first. Yet, like any skill, it becomes more intuitive over time. The initial strictness of the elimination phase of the diet eases into the more flexible and personal phase of reintroduction. This phase is where the real magic happens, as you begin to tailor the low FODMAP guidelines to fit your lifestyle and preferences, creating a customized approach that allows for maximum health with minimum restriction.

In essence, learning to recognize high and low FODMAP foods isn't just about dietary limitations it's about expanding your culinary horizons within a new framework. This new dietary language not only improves communication between you and your body but also between you and the larger world of culinary delights. It provides a foundation not just for symptom management, but for a deeper, more joyful engagement with the nourishing possibilities of food.

2.3 TAILORING THE DIET TO YOUR SPECIFIC NEEDS

While understanding the basic principles of the low-FODMAP diet is crucial, the true craftsmanship lies in tailoring these guidelines to suit your unique dietary needs and lifestyle. This is not about following a one-size-fits-all approach; rather, it's about sculpting a dietary plan that molds seamlessly into the contours of your daily life and personal health requirements.

Transforming a generalized eating plan into your personalized nutritional guide involves several steps, each as crucial as the last, all centered around the core principle: listening intently to your body's messages. Embarking on this adaptive journey can be likened to being a chef in your kitchen where instincts, attention to detail, and adaptability lead to the creation of dishes that are not only safe but also delightful and nourishing.

Firstly, it's imperative to start with a clean slate, commonly referred to as the elimination phase. This initial stage is where you carefully remove high FODMAP foods from your diet, which often feels like stripping back the layers of an intricate painting to reveal the blank canvas beneath. This process is vital as it sets the baseline from which you can start identifying triggers and adapting your diet.

As you navigate through this phase, it's essential to maintain a detailed food diary. This diary should go beyond simply logging what you eat; it should also record how you feel after each meal. Are you bloated, experiencing discomfort, or feeling just fine? These notes become invaluable data, painting a clear picture of how specific foods interact with your digestive system.

Transitioning into the reintroduction phase, your diary plays a crucial role. Here, you begin to reintroduce high FODMAP foods one at a time, like an artist adding color slowly back to the canvas, observing how each shade interacts with the overall picture. This controlled, methodical process allows you to pinpoint which foods provoke symptoms, and importantly, which do not, enabling you to add tolerable foods back into your diet and expand your culinary repertoire.

This phase not only uncovers food intolerances but also helps in determining portion sizes that your body can handle, which might be just as critical. The FODMAP threshold varies from person to person and even from one food to another. You might find, for instance, that while a half cup of cooked pasta sits well, a full cup triggers symptoms. Understanding these nuances is key to customizing your diet without feeling deprived.

Once you have identified your personal triggers and tolerable foods and portions, the next step is learning to maintain this tailored diet in the long-term integrating it sustainably into your lifestyle. This means finding ways to incorporate a variety of low FODMAP foods that you enjoy, to ensure nutritional balance and prevent dietary boredom.

Moreover, the need for adaptability extends beyond the home. Dining out, traveling, and celebrating special occasions all require applying what you've learned about your dietary needs in different contexts. Building self-advocacy skills, such as requesting specific preparations of food when dining out or explaining your dietary restrictions to hosts, becomes part of your toolkit.

In this customizing process, external support can also be immensely beneficial. Working with a dietitian who specializes in the low-FODMAP diet can provide you with tailored advice and adjustments based on your ongoing experiences and symptoms. They can help fine-tune your diet to better suit changes in lifestyle, health status, or even goals such as weight management or addressing nutritional deficiencies.

Consider the case of Michael, a freelance graphic designer with a predilection for culinary experimentation. He discovered through his reintroduction phase that he could handle certain oligosaccharides in moderation, something he wouldn't have risked without the structured approach of the low-FODMAP diet. With clever tweaks and creative culinary substitutes, his diet became both a palette for his artistry and a foundation for his well-being, illustrating the profound personalization possible with this approach.

Ultimately, transforming the low-FODMAP diet to meet your specific needs is about creating harmony between your health requirements and your enjoyment of life. It's about turning dietary boundaries into avenues for exploration, ensuring each meal not only nourishes your body but also brings joy to your palate. This tailored approach doesn't just aim to manage symptoms; it strives to enhance your quality of life, making the diet a tailor-made suit designed to fit perfectly and comfortably, enabling you to live your life to the fullest.

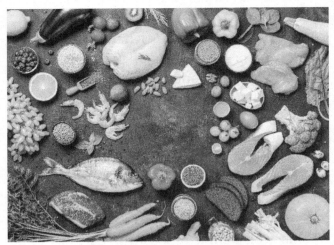

Navigating the world of dietary choices can often feel like uncharted territory, but a well-informed guidebook in hand can turn those bewildering maps into clear paths. That's precisely what we aim to provide in this chapter a detailed food guide tailored for those following a Low-FODMAP diet. Understanding what to include on your plate and what to avoid can make all the difference in managing digestive health issues and enjoying daily meals without fear.

Imagine stepping into your local grocery store armed with the knowledge of exactly what nourishes your body and what could potentially trigger your symptoms. It's empowering, isn't it? Here, we dissect the complex world of food ingredients, starting from the staples that fill your pantry and fridge to interpreting the often-puzzling labels that adorn packaged foods.

The key to thriving on a Low-FODMAP diet is not just about avoiding high-FODMAP foods; it's about replacing them with equally nutritious and satisfying alternatives. Picture this: you're planning your meals for the week. Where you might once have felt restricted by the ingredients you should avoid, now, you can find comfort and creativity in the array of foods you can include. A crisp salad of mixed greens tossed with juicy orange segments, sprinkled with seeds, and drizzled with a homemade dressing it's not only doable, but it's also delicious and safe on this diet.

Furthermore, to assist you in making these decisions swiftly and confidently, we'll delve into understanding how to interpret food labels effectively. This knowledge acts as a shield, protecting you from the hidden FODMAPs that often lurk in processed foods, enabling you to make informed choices swiftly, even during hurried shopping trips.

This chapter is your compass and map rolled into one, pointing you towards food choices that promise not only to keep symptoms at bay but also to enrich your culinary journey, ensuring it remains as flavorful as it is hearty and healthful. Let's begin this journey with confidence and curiosity, ready to explore the bountiful options that align with your health goals and palate.

3.1 FOODS TO INCLUDE AND EXCLUDE

When embarking on the Low-FODMAP diet, the decision about what to eat and what to avoid is akin to learning a new language. It's about understanding which foods bring comfort and health, and which might trigger an adverse reaction it's a personal journey of discovery and adjustment.

While it's crucial to know the lengthy lists of what to include and eat, an equally important aspect, often overlooked, is the sense of freedom and control restored by learning how to navigate these choices. This journey of culinary discovery opens up a new realm of possibilities that, despite initial perceptions, are rich with variety and flavor.

Let's begin with what many might consider the cornerstone of any diet the staples. These include proteins, fruits, vegetables, grains, and dairy products. For those managing digestive sensitivities, focusing on these categories in their safe forms is crucial.

Proteins

Proteins are vital, yet, navigating proteins on a Low-FODMAP diet initially seems limiting. However, most unprocessed meats and fish are FODMAP free. The key here is simplicity grilled chicken breast, pan-seared salmon, or even a succulent beef steak are not only safe but also provide a canvas for experimenting with various Low-FODMAP herbs and spices. The risk typically lies in processed meats like sausages or meatballs, often laden with onion, garlic, or other high-FODMAP fillers. Opting for simplicity not only ensures safety but also helps highlight the natural flavors of these proteins.

Vegetables

Vegetables represent a dichotomy in the Low-FODMAP world. On one hand, there are numerous vegetables like carrots, eggplant, potatoes, and bell peppers that are excellent choices. They provide not just essential nutrients but also diversity in texture and flavor to dishes. On the other hand, there are also high-FODMAP choices such as onions and garlic, staples in many kitchens, which are famously problematic. However, the introduction of garlic-infused oils and the clever use of chives or the green parts of spring onions provides that beloved flavor without the FODMAPs.

Fruits

Fruits often strike fear into the hearts of those starting a Low-FODMAP diet, as so many beloved options are off-limits. Apples, pears, and cherries might step back, but this paves the way for others to shine. Oranges, grapes, strawberries, and blueberries are not only safe but are also rich in vitamins, offering sweet fixes without the fructose overload. Think of a blueberry smoothie or a strawberry-topped oatmeal options that keep breakfast both colorful and comforting.

Grains

Grains often form the backbone of meals, yet navigating them can be tricky. While wheat, barley, and rye are out, there are numerous Low-FODMAP grains that can take center stage. Quinoa, rice, and oats are excellent alternatives that not only satisfy the need for substantial, comforting carbs but also provide a fantastic nutritional profile. These grains can become the base for a hearty breakfast porridge or a filling dinner side, adding both substance and variety to meals.

Dairy and Alternatives

Dairy loved for its creaminess and rich flavor often poses a conundrum. Lactose, the primary carbohydrate in dairy products, is a major FODMAP. However, not all dairy needs to be forbidden. Hard cheeses like cheddar, and lactose-free milk or yogurts, can safely find their way back into your fridge. They allow the richness of dairy to be enjoyed imagine a sprinkle of parmesan over a freshly tossed salad or a dollop of lactose-free yogurt on a baked potato.

Understanding food labels is as crucial as knowing the foods themselves. Hidden FODMAPs are a common pitfall, so learning to decipher labels can liberate and prevent unintended symptoms. For instance, additives like inulin, a common fiber supplement in processed foods, could cause flare-ups. Acquainting oneself with such terms protects and educates.

The art of substitution is invaluable. It's about re-imaging meals with a unique twist using polenta instead of a wheat-based side dish, or garnishing with green onion tops instead of white onions. These swaps not only keep meals exciting and varied but ensure they are safe, aligning with both health needs and culinary pleasure.

Far from the restrictive diet it might seem, the Low-FODMAP diet opens up a new perspective on food, focusing on what can be included rather than what must be excluded. It encourages a return to whole, unprocessed foods, which inherently simplifies and enriches the diet. Each safe ingredient offers a step towards symptom control, but more importantly, it contributes to a broader canvas on which to paint your dietary landscape, rich with flavor, color, and texture. Embarking on this journey isn't just about avoiding discomfort but rediscovering pleasure in meals, ensuring every dish is as delightful as it is safe. This understanding not only facilitates a smoother transition into the diet but enhances life quality, proving that dietary restrictions don't have to mean culinary restrictions.

3.2 SIMPLE SUBSTITUTIONS FOR EVERYDAY USE

In the realm of cooking on a Low-FODMAP diet, the act of substitution is not merely a tactic, but an art form, a creative endeavor that allows for the reinvention of beloved dishes without trigger ingredients. The beauty of substitutions lies in their ability to transform a meal from a potential risk to a gut-friendly delight, ensuring both peace of mind and pleasure.

Consider the usual staples in your pantry and refrigerator. Certain ingredients, while seemingly benign, could be the very culprits of discomfort. However, with a few clever tweaks to these everyday items, one can still relish the flavors of a full, rich diet. Making these adjustments can be quite simple with a foundational knowledge of suitable alternatives.

The Challenge with Staples

Take onions and garlic, for example, which are almost ubiquitous in cuisines worldwide. Their pungent flavors and aromas are nearly irreplaceable in stirring up the base essences of countless dishes. Yet, for someone on a Low-FODMAP diet, these are among the first items that need to be moderated. Fortunately, the solution doesn't lie far. The green parts of scallions or leeks can impart a similar depth and pungency to dishes. For garlic, infusing oils with its essence provides the beloved flavor without the fructans responsible for digestive distress.

Reimagining Dairy

In the dairy aisle, where lactose lurks around every corner, the switch to lactose-free products is a straightforward one. Lactose-free milk, cheese, and yogurt are processed to remove lactose, making them gentle on the gut without compromising on taste or texture. For those who prefer plant-based alternatives, almond milk, coconut yogurt, and aged cheeses such as Parmesan, which naturally contains little to no lactose, are excellent choices. Each of these offers versatility in both cooking and direct consumption.

Bread and Cereal Swaps

Bread, a staple in many diets, typically contains wheat and thereby fructans. However, the availability of gluten-free bread made without wheat, barley, or rye presents a viable alternative. These products are often crafted with rice flour, potato starch, or other gluten-free grains that fit well within the Low-FODMAP regimen. Similarly, breakfast cereals can be replaced with oats or quinoa flakes, which provide an excellent start to the day without unnecessary fructans.

Redefining Sweetness

When it comes to sweetening agents, the challenge is twofold. Not only is it about avoiding high fructose corn syrup, but also managing natural sources rich in fructans and polyols, such as honey and agave. Thankfully, pure maple syrup and granulated sugar are free of FODMAPs, offering the sweet touch needed in desserts or beverages without the adverse effects.

Adapting Sauces and Condiments

Sauces and condiments are another hidden harbor of high FODMAP ingredients. Soy sauce and traditional pasta sauces can be replaced with tamari and homemade tomato sauce seasoned with low-FODMAP herbs. Instead of store-bought salad dressings, a simple dressing using olive oil, vinegar, mustard, and herbs can elevate salads without inducing symptoms.

Cooking Oils and Fats

When considering oils and fats, the focus is less about FODMAPs since fats and oils don't contain carbs and more about overall health. Opt for oils with a high smoke point for cooking, such as olive oil or canola oil, which provide the necessary fat content for cooking without health risks associated with saturated fats.

Snack Modifications

Finally, for snacking, nuts and seeds are a preferred option, but it's essential to choose varieties that are Low-FODMAP friendly. Almonds, peanuts, and pumpkin seeds make great choices in moderation. Replacing high-FODMAP snacks like garlic-flavored crisps or cashews with these alternatives can help maintain a healthy digestive system.

In transforming these staples through simple substitutions, one discovers not only the feasibility of maintaining a diverse and appealing diet but also the potential for new culinary favorites to emerge. These adaptations are not merely about restriction but about reconceptualizing the approach to food an approach that embraces variety, taste, and health in equal measure.

By mastering the art of substitution, you empower yourself to cook with confidence and creativity. This process turns the kitchen from a place of dietary limitations into a canvas for culinary creativity, where every meal serves as a testament to a personalized, sensitive diet that is as rich in variety as it is in flavor. Hence, embracing these substitutions makes the process of cooking and eating a more enjoyable, accessible, and symptom-free experience.

3.3 INTERPRETING FOOD LABELS FOR FODMAP CONTENT

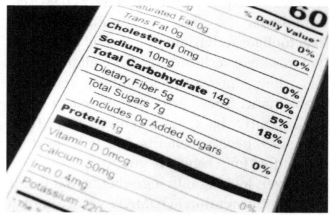

Embarking on the Low-FODMAP journey brings its own set of challenges, and one of the trickiest can be navigating the grocery store aisles specifically, interpreting food labels. For those with digestive sensitivities, the supermarket can sometimes seem like a minefield scattered with hidden FODMAPs in ingredients lists that are anything but straightforward.

Understanding food labels is a skill that can demystify the shopping process and arm you with knowledge to make empowered choices. As you stand in the grocery store, scanning various products, it's not just about avoiding obvious offenders like wheat or dairy. Many ingredients that are high in FODMAPs are not so easily recognizable and can lurk under names that are unfamiliar.

When you look at a food label, the first thing to note is the serving size, which sets the stage for understanding how much of each nutrient, including sugars and fiber, you'll be consuming based on the quantity you eat. The key is not just looking for "sugar" as an ingredient but identifying other names it might hide under, such as high fructose corn syrup, agave nectar, honey, or even more obscure names like sorbitol, mannitol, and xylitol. These are sugar alcohols that can be particularly troublesome for those with IBS or similar gastrointestinal sensitivities.

Turning your attention to the fiber content, while dietary fiber is beneficial, not all fibers are created equal in the world of FODMAPs. Ingredients like inulin, FOS (fructooligosaccharides), and GOS (galactooligosaccharides), although promoted for their prebiotic qualities, can be problematic. These are often added to foods like yogurt, bars, and snacks for their supposed health benefits but can lead to discomfort for a sensitive gut.

Moreover, looking into ingredients that might not directly mention FODMAPs yet are known sources can save much distress. For example, anything containing lactose, whey protein concentrate (not isolate, which is fine), or milk solids should be approached with caution. Similarly, additives like maltodextrin, although not a FODMAP per se, can still cause digestive issues for some people.

The complexity increases as certain foods contain both low and high-FODMAP ingredients. Take a bottle of salad dressing, for example. You might see olive oil and lemon juice (both low-FODMAP) listed alongside garlic and honey (high-FODMAP). In these cases, evaluating your personal tolerances becomes key. Knowledge of which ingredients can be digested comfortably allows you to make informed decisions about which products to put back on the shelf and which to take home.

As you become more familiar with these terms, you start to recognize patterns and common culprits, making your shopping experiences quicker and more confident. There are even dedicated applications and guides designed to help decode these labels with ease, turning what could be a taxing process into a breezy supermarket stroll.

Understanding food labels also means knowing technicalities used in food manufacturing. For instance, "natural flavors" can be a confusing term, as it could essentially mean anything derived from a natural source, including onion or garlic derivatives. Here, reaching out to manufacturers to confirm ingredients can be worthwhile when in doubt. The journey through each aisle can be simplified by planning ahead. Creating a list of "safe" brands or products, maintaining a diary of personal trigger ingredients, and even familiarizing oneself with FODMAP-friendly certifications can streamline the process. Many products now boast labels indicating they are FODMAP-friendly, a testament to the growing recognition of dietary needs and a boon for those following this diet.

Integrating these strategies into your shopping routine doesn't just reduce the physical symptoms but also alleviates the mental strain that can come from trying to make safe dietary choices. It restores a sense of normalcy and control over your diet and your health, transforming grocery shopping from a daunting task into an enjoyable activity.

Ultimately, the art of interpreting food labels is about more than avoiding discomfort; it's about embracing an informed way of living that aligns with your health goals and culinary practices. With each product you place in your cart, you're reinforcing your commitment to a healthier, happier gut. It's here, amidst the grocery store aisles, that your empowerment and your journey towards improved well-being truly begins.

CHAPTER 4: COMPLETE FOOD LIST

LOW FODMAP-FRIENDLY INGREDIENTS

1. Fruits (Low in FODMAPs):

- Bananas (ripe)
- Strawberries
- Blueberries
- Raspberries
- Oranges
- Grapes (red, green)
- Kiwi
- Pineapple
- Cantaloupe (rockmelon)
- Honeydew melon
- Dragon fruit (pitaya)
- Papaya
- Lemon
- Lime
- Rhubarb

2. Vegetables (Low in FODMAPs):

- Spinach (baby and regular)
- Carrots
- Zucchini (courgette)
- Bell peppers (capsicum)
- Cucumber
- Lettuce (iceberg, butter, romaine)
- Tomato (common, cherry, grape)
- Eggplant (aubergine)
- Green beans
- Alfalfa sprouts
- Swiss chard (silverbeet)
- Kale (in small amounts)
- Bok choy (pak choi)
- Radish
- Turnip
- Collard greens
- Fennel leaves (fronds)
- Chives
- Olives
- Parsnips
- Potatoes (regular and sweet in small portions)

3. Grains, Starches, and Cereals:

- White rice
- Brown rice
- Quinoa
- Oats (plain, gluten-free)
- Cornmeal (polenta)
- Millet
- Buckwheat
- Tapioca
- Gluten-free bread (check ingredients)
- Gluten-free pasta (rice, quinoa-based)
- Rice cakes
- Rice noodles

4. Dairy and Dairy Substitutes:

- Lactose-free milk (cow, goat)
- Lactose-free yogurt (plain or flavored)
- Hard cheeses (cheddar, parmesan, pecorino, swiss)
- Lactose-free soft cheeses (brie, camembert, cream cheese in small amounts)
- Almond milk (unsweetened)
- Coconut milk (canned, small amounts)
- Coconut yogurt (without high FODMAP ingredients)
- Butter (lactose-free or regular in small quantities)
- Ghee (clarified butter)

5. Protein (Meat, Fish, Poultry, and Vegetarian Sources):

- Chicken (no seasoning with garlic/onion)
- Turkey
- Beef (unprocessed)
- Pork (unprocessed)
- Lamb
- Fish (salmon, tuna, cod, sardines, etc.)
- Shellfish (shrimp, lobster, crab, mussels)
- Eggs
- Firm tofu (not silken tofu)
- Tempeh
- Quorn (check ingredients)

6. Legumes and Pulses (allowed in small portions):

- Canned lentils (rinsed thoroughly, in small amounts)
- Canned chickpeas (rinsed thoroughly, in small amounts)

7. Nuts and Seeds (Low FODMAP in moderation):

- Almonds (10-12 nuts per serving)
- Macadamia nuts
- Pecans
- Peanuts
- Walnuts
- Pine nuts
- Chia seeds
- Flaxseeds (linseeds)
- Pumpkin seeds
- Sesame seeds
- Sunflower seeds

8. Oils, Fats, and Butter:

- Olive oil (regular and garlic-infused)
- Coconut oil
- Sunflower oil
- Canola oil
- Garlic-infused oil (without garlic pieces)
- Butter (lactose-free or regular in moderation)
- Ghee

9. Herbs and Spices:

- Basil
- Parsley
- Coriander (cilantro)
- Oregano
- Thyme
- Rosemary
- Mint
- Dill
- Chives
- Ginger
- Turmeric
- Paprika
- Cumin
- Cinnamon
- Bay leaves
- Lemon zest
- Pepper (black, white)

10. Sweeteners:

- Maple syrup (pure, not with added fructose)
- Sugar (in small amounts)
- Rice malt syrup
- Stevia

11. Beverages:

- Coffee (in moderation)
- Tea (black, green, peppermint)
- Herbal teas (chamomile and fennel in small amounts)
- Water (sparkling or still)
- Lactose-free milk or dairy substitutes

12. Snacks:

- Plain popcorn (without garlic/onion powder)
- Rice cakes (plain or lightly salted)
- Gluten-free crackers (check for added FODMAPs)
- Corn chips (plain)

- Seaweed snacks
- Homemade low-FODMAP granola

13. Flours (Low FODMAP for baking):

- Rice flour
- Quinoa flour
- Corn flour (cornstarch)
- Potato flour
- Tapioca flour
- Almond flour (in moderation)
- Buckwheat flour
- Coconut flour (in small amounts)

HIGH FODMAP INGREDIENTS TO AVOID

1. Fruits (high in FODMAPs):

- Apples
- Pears
- Mango
- Watermelon
- Cherries
- Plums
- Peaches
- Apricots
- Nectarines
- Blackberries
- Figs (fresh and dried)
- Dates
- Prunes
- Grapes (in large quantities)
- Pomegranate
- Papaya (in large quantities)
- Dried fruits (raisins, cranberries with added sugars)

2. Vegetables (high in FODMAPs):

- Garlic (including garlic powder)
- Onion (including onion powder)
- Shallots
- Leeks (white part)
- Spring onions (white part)
- Asparagus
- Cauliflower
- Broccoli (large portions, especially stems)
- Brussels sprouts
- Cabbage (savoy, napa, red, white)
- Mushrooms (all varieties, including button, portobello, shiitake)
- Artichokes
- Snow peas
- Sugar snap peas
- Beetroot (in large amounts)
- Celery (more than 1/4 stalk)
- Fennel bulb
- Okra

3. Legumes and pulses (high in FODMAPs):

- Chickpeas (whole or dry)
- Lentils (dry)
- Kidney beans
- Black beans
- Borlotti beans
- Soybeans
- Navy beans
- Split peas
- Mung beans
- Edamame (fresh soybeans)

4. Grains and cereals (high in FODMAPs):

- Wheat (including whole wheat, white, and spelt)
- Rye
- Barley
- Couscous
- Bulgur wheat
- Semolina
- Farro
- Bran (wheat bran, oat bran)
- Regular bread made with wheat, rye, or barley
- Regular pasta (made from wheat, rye, or barley)
- Cereals made from wheat or rye (wheat-based breakfast cereals, muesli, granola with added wheat or inulin)

5. Dairy (high in lactose):

- Cow's milk
- Goat's milk
- Sheep's milk
- Regular yogurt (cow, sheep, or goat)
- Ice cream (made with regular milk or cream)

- Fresh and soft cheeses (ricotta, mascarpone, cream cheese, cottage cheese, feta, brie, camembert in large amounts)
- Sour cream
- Milk-based creams (whipped cream, heavy cream)
- Buttermilk

6. Nuts and seeds (high in FODMAPs):

- Pistachios
- Cashews

7. Sweeteners and syrups (high in FODMAPs):

- Honey (high in fructose)
- High-fructose corn syrup (HFCS)
- Agave syrup
- Sorbitol (E420) – found in sugar-free candies and gum
- Mannitol (E421)
- Xylitol (E967)
- Maltitol (E965)
- Isomalt (E953)

8. Processed and packaged foods (with hidden FODMAPs):

- Packaged foods with garlic or onion powder (like chips, sauces, and marinades)
- Pre-made soups with garlic, onion, or wheat thickeners
- Snack bars with high-FODMAP fruits, inulin, or honey
- Gluten-free products containing high-FODMAP ingredients like soy flour or chicory root (inulin)
- Sauces and dressings containing onion, garlic, honey, or high-fructose corn syrup
- Canned beans (unless thoroughly rinsed and used in small quantities)

9. Beverages:

- Milk-based drinks (e.g., milkshakes, smoothies with regular milk or yogurt)
- Fruit juices made from high FODMAP fruits (e.g., apple juice, pear juice, mango juice)
- Coconut water (in large amounts)
- Beer (in large amounts, due to malt from barley)
- Rum (high in polyols)
- Certain fortified wines like port and sherry

10. Meat and meat products (with added FODMAPs):

- Processed meats containing onion, garlic, or wheat fillers (e.g., sausages, meatballs)
- Marinated meats with high FODMAP ingredients (onion, garlic, soy sauce with wheat)

11. Condiments and sauces:

- Ketchup (in large amounts, due to high fructose corn syrup or onion/garlic)
- BBQ sauce (due to onion, garlic, or high fructose corn syrup)
- Soy sauce (in large quantities, especially if made with wheat)
- Chutneys (containing apple, mango, or dried fruits)
- Relish (due to added onion and garlic)
- Marinades with onion or garlic
- Pesto (if made with garlic)
- Hummus (due to chickpeas and garlic)

12. Herbs, spices, and flavor enhancers:

- Garlic (fresh, dried, or powdered)
- Onion (fresh, dried, or powdered)
- Shallots
- Asafoetida (unless used in very small amounts)
- Certain pre-made spice blends (check for added garlic, onion, or wheat)

13. Dried and processed fruits (high in FODMAPs):

- Raisins
- Dried apricots
- Dried figs
- Dried dates
- Dried prunes
- Dried apples
- Dried pears

14. Baked goods:

- Pastries, cakes, and cookies made with wheat flour, honey, or high fructose corn syrup
- Muffins and cupcakes containing high-FODMAP fruits or wheat flour
- Donuts, croissants, and pies made with regular flour

Chapter 5: Breakfast Delights

Mornings can often be a hurried affair, especially if you're navigating the complexities of a low-FODMAP diet. However, with a little creativity and planning, breakfast can transform from a quick, forgettable necessity into a delightful, nourishing start to your day. In this chapter, we explore the realm of breakfast delights that not only comply with your dietary needs but also infuse joy and variety into your morning ritual.

Imagine the comfort of warm, soothing meals greeting you at the dawn, or the refreshing zest of fruity bowls that wake up your taste buds. This image is not just a dream but a tangible reality with a low-FODMAP regimen. The art of breakfast, within the confines of dietary restrictions, doesn't have to be bland or boring. Instead, it's an opportunity to be innovative with the ingredients that nourish your body and respect its needs.

In crafting these breakfast recipes, I tapped into the quiet magic of mornings those moments when the world seems to pause and the kitchen becomes a sanctuary. A steaming plate of oat pancakes, made from gluten-free oats and topped with a homemade strawberry compote, can make the first meal of the day feel like a celebration rather than a chore. Or, consider a smooth blend of lactose-free yogurt with swirls of maple syrup and sprinkles of toasted walnuts and chia seeds for a quick yet luxurious eating experience.

The recipes in this chapter are designed to be both functional and indulgent. They acknowledge the hectic pace of morning routines while offering you the tools to prepare quick, satisfying meals. From hearty, savory dishes that can be cooked in bulk and enjoyed throughout the week, to sweet, instant treats ready in minutes, each recipe is aimed at easing your morning routine without compromising on flavor or your dietary needs. So, let's bring enjoyment back to your morning meal with delicious, gut-friendly breakfast options that keep your kitchen inspiring and your mornings serene. Here's to starting the day right, embracing the possibilities of the low-FODMAP diet, and nourishing not just your body but also your spirit with every bite.

AVOCADO & SPINACH BREAKFAST SMOOTHIE

PREPARATION TIME: 5 min
COOKING TIME: 0 min
MODE OF COOKING: Blending
SERVINGS: 2
INGREDIENTS:

- 1 ripe avocado, pitted and peeled
- 1 cup baby spinach leaves, packed
- 1 banana, frozen
- 1 Tbsp chia seeds
- 1/2 cup lactose-free plain yogurt
- 1 cup almond milk, unsweetened
- 1 tsp maple syrup (optional)
- 1/2 tsp vanilla extract

DIRECTIONS:

1. Add all ingredients to a blender.
2. Blend on high until smooth and creamy.
3. Pour into glasses and serve immediately.

TIPS:

- Add a handful of ice cubes for a colder, thicker smoothie.
- Substitute spinach with kale for a different flavor profile.

N.V.: Calories: 250, Fat: 15g, Carbs: 28g, Protein: 5g, Sugar: 12g, Sodium: 80mg, Potassium: 740mg, Cholesterol: 0mg

QUICK QUINOA BREAKFAST BOWL

PREPARATION TIME: 5 min
COOKING TIME: 15 min
MODE OF COOKING: Stovetop
SERVINGS: 2
INGREDIENTS:

- 1/2 cup quinoa, rinsed
- 1 cup water
- 1/4 cup lactose-free milk
- 1 Tbsp almond butter
- 1 Tbsp maple syrup
- 1/2 tsp cinnamon
- 1/4 cup blueberries
- 1/4 cup sliced almonds

DIRECTIONS:

1. In a small saucepan, bring quinoa and water to a boil.
2. Reduce heat, cover, and simmer for 15 min, or until water is absorbed.
3. Fluff quinoa with a fork and stir in lactose-free milk, almond butter, maple syrup, and cinnamon.
4. Divide between two bowls and top with blueberries and sliced almonds.

TIPS:

- Substitute almond butter with peanut butter for a different taste.
- Use any seasonal fruit for topping.

N.V.: Calories: 320, Fat: 13g, Carbs: 42g, Protein: 10g, Sugar: 10g, Sodium: 50mg, Potassium: 450mg, Cholesterol: 0mg

SCRAMBLED EGGS WITH SPINACH AND FETA

PREPARATION TIME: 5 min
COOKING TIME: 5 min
MODE OF COOKING: Stovetop
SERVINGS: 2
INGREDIENTS:

- 4 large eggs
- 1/4 cup lactose-free milk
- 1/2 cup baby spinach, chopped
- 1/4 cup feta cheese, crumbled (low-FODMAP)
- 1 Tbsp olive oil
- Salt and pepper to taste

DIRECTIONS:

1. In a bowl, whisk together eggs and lactose-free milk.
2. Heat olive oil in a non-stick skillet over medium heat.
3. Add spinach to the skillet and sauté until wilted, about 1-2 min.
4. Pour egg mixture into the skillet, stirring gently to scramble.
5. Once eggs are nearly cooked, add feta and cook until eggs are fully set.

6. Season with salt and pepper before serving.

TIPS:
- Serve with a slice of gluten-free toast for a complete meal.
- Add a pinch of turmeric for added health benefits.

N.V.: Calories: 250, Fat: 19g, Carbs: 4g, Protein: 16g, Sugar: 2g, Sodium: 360mg, Potassium: 300mg, Cholesterol: 385mg

BANANA OAT PANCAKES

PREPARATION TIME: 5 min
COOKING TIME: 10 min
MODE OF COOKING: Stovetop
SERVINGS: 2
INGREDIENTS:
- 1 ripe banana, mashed
- 1/2 cup gluten-free rolled oats
- 1/4 cup lactose-free milk
- 1 large egg
- 1/2 tsp baking powder
- 1/2 tsp vanilla extract
- 1/2 tsp cinnamon
- 1 Tbsp coconut oil

DIRECTIONS:
1. In a bowl, mix together mashed banana, oats, milk, egg, baking powder, vanilla, and cinnamon.
2. Heat coconut oil in a non-stick skillet over medium heat.
3. Pour 1/4 cup of batter onto the skillet for each pancake.
4. Cook until bubbles form on the surface, then flip and cook the other side until golden brown.
5. Serve warm with a drizzle of maple syrup if desired.

TIPS:
- Add chopped nuts or seeds for extra texture.
- Use a blender to smooth the batter for a finer texture.

N.V.: Calories: 320, Fat: 12g, Carbs: 46g, Protein: 8g, Sugar: 12g, Sodium: 180mg, Potassium: 450mg, Cholesterol: 70mg

VEGGIE-PACKED OMELET

PREPARATION TIME: 5 min
COOKING TIME: 10 min
MODE OF COOKING: Stovetop
SERVINGS: 1
INGREDIENTS:
- 2 large eggs
- 1/4 cup lactose-free milk
- 1/4 cup zucchini, grated
- 1/4 cup bell pepper, diced
- 1/4 cup cherry tomatoes, halved
- 1 Tbsp fresh parsley, chopped
- 1 Tbsp olive oil
- Salt and pepper to taste

DIRECTIONS:
1. In a bowl, whisk eggs and milk until well combined.
2. Heat olive oil in a non-stick skillet over medium heat.
3. Add zucchini, bell pepper, and cherry tomatoes to the skillet, sauté for 3-4 min until softened.
4. Pour egg mixture over the vegetables and cook until edges begin to set.
5. Fold the omelet in half and continue to cook until eggs are fully set.
6. Sprinkle with fresh parsley before serving.

TIPS:
- Substitute zucchini with spinach for a different flavor.
- Add a sprinkle of cheese if desired.

N.V.: Calories: 220, Fat: 17g, Carbs: 5g, Protein: 12g, Sugar: 4g, Sodium: 170mg, Potassium: 450mg, Cholesterol: 330mg

SIMPLE OATMEAL WITH STRAWBERRIES

PREPARATION TIME: 5 min
COOKING TIME: 10 min
MODE OF COOKING: Stovetop
SERVINGS: 2
INGREDIENTS:
- 1 cup gluten-free rolled oats
- 2 cups water or lactose-free milk

- 1 Tbsp maple syrup (optional)
- 1/2 cup fresh strawberries, sliced
- 1/4 tsp cinnamon

DIRECTIONS:

1. In a medium saucepan, bring water or lactose-free milk to a boil.
2. Stir in the gluten-free rolled oats and reduce heat to low. Simmer for 5-7 min, stirring occasionally, until the oats are tender.
3. Stir in the maple syrup (if using) and cinnamon.
4. Divide the oatmeal into bowls and top with fresh strawberries.
5. Serve warm.

TIPS:

- Add a handful of blueberries for extra flavor.
- Top with a sprinkle of lactose-free granola for added crunch.

N.V.: Calories: 220, Fat: 4g, Carbs: 42g, Protein: 6g, Sugar: 10g, Sodium: 10mg, Potassium: 150mg, Cholesterol: 0mg

BERRY QUINOA BREAKFAST BOWL

PREPARATION TIME: 10 min
COOKING TIME: 15 min
MODE OF COOKING: Stovetop
SERVINGS: 2
INGREDIENTS:

- 1/2 cup quinoa, rinsed
- 1 cup water
- 1/4 cup lactose-free milk
- 1 Tbsp maple syrup
- 1/2 tsp vanilla extract
- 1/2 cup mixed berries (blueberries, raspberries, strawberries)
- 1 Tbsp chia seeds
- 1/4 cup sliced almonds
- Fresh mint leaves for garnish (optional)

DIRECTIONS:

1. In a small saucepan, combine quinoa and water. Bring to a boil.

2. Reduce heat, cover, and simmer for 15 min, or until the water is absorbed and quinoa is tender.
3. Fluff quinoa with a fork and stir in lactose-free milk, maple syrup, and vanilla extract.
4. Divide quinoa between two bowls. Top with mixed berries, chia seeds, and sliced almonds.
5. Garnish with fresh mint leaves, if desired, and serve warm.

TIPS:

- Substitute berries with seasonal fruits for variety.
- Add a sprinkle of cinnamon for extra flavor.

N.V.: Calories: 320, Fat: 11g, Carbs: 50g, Protein: 9g, Sugar: 16g, Sodium: 35mg, Potassium: 350mg, Cholesterol: 0mg

SAVORY OATMEAL WITH SPINACH AND EGG

PREPARATION TIME: 5 min
COOKING TIME: 10 min
MODE OF COOKING: Stovetop
SERVINGS: 2
INGREDIENTS:

- 1 cup gluten-free rolled oats
- 2 cups water or lactose-free milk
- 1 cup fresh spinach, chopped
- 2 large eggs
- 1 Tbsp olive oil
- Salt and pepper to taste
- 1/4 tsp smoked paprika (optional)

DIRECTIONS:

1. In a medium saucepan, bring the water or lactose-free milk to a boil. Add the gluten-free oats, reduce heat, and simmer for 5-7 min until the oats are tender.
2. While the oats are cooking, heat olive oil in a non-stick skillet over medium heat. Add the chopped spinach and sauté until wilted, about 2 min.

3. In the same skillet, fry the eggs until the whites are set and the yolks are cooked to your liking.
4. Divide the cooked oatmeal into two bowls. Top each with sautéed spinach and a fried egg.
5. Season with salt, pepper, and smoked paprika if using. Serve immediately.

TIPS:
- Add a sprinkle of lactose-free cheese for extra flavor.
- Top with avocado slices for a more filling meal.

N.V.: Calories: 320, Fat: 14g, Carbs: 38g, Protein: 14g, Sugar: 1g, Sodium: 120mg, Potassium: 450mg, Cholesterol: 185mg

SWEET POTATO AND AVOCADO BREAKFAST BOWL

PREPARATION TIME: 10 min
COOKING TIME: 20 min
MODE OF COOKING: Stovetop
SERVINGS: 2
INGREDIENTS:
- 1 medium sweet potato, peeled and cubed
- 1 ripe avocado, sliced
- 2 large eggs
- 1 Tbsp olive oil
- Salt and pepper to taste
- 1/4 tsp smoked paprika (optional)

DIRECTIONS:
1. Boil the sweet potato cubes in a pot of water for 10-12 min, or until tender. Drain and set aside.
2. In a non-stick skillet, heat olive oil over medium heat. Fry the eggs to your desired doneness.
3. Divide the sweet potato cubes between two bowls. Top each with sliced avocado and a fried egg.
4. Season with salt, pepper, and smoked paprika if using. Serve immediately.

TIPS:
- Add a sprinkle of chopped fresh herbs like cilantro or parsley.

- Serve with a side of gluten-free toast for a more filling meal.

N.V.: Calories: 350, Fat: 24g, Carbs: 28g, Protein: 9g, Sugar: 4g, Sodium: 180mg, Potassium: 700mg, Cholesterol: 185mg

WARM CINNAMON QUINOA PORRIDGE

PREPARATION TIME: 5 min
COOKING TIME: 15 min
MODE OF COOKING: Stovetop
SERVINGS: 2
INGREDIENTS:
- 1/2 cup quinoa, rinsed
- 1 cup lactose-free milk or water
- 1/2 tsp ground cinnamon
- 1 Tbsp maple syrup (optional)
- 1/4 cup chopped pecans
- 1/4 cup fresh or dried cranberries

DIRECTIONS:
1. In a small saucepan, bring the lactose-free milk or water to a boil. Add the rinsed quinoa, reduce heat, cover, and simmer for 15 min or until the quinoa is tender and the liquid is absorbed.
2. Stir in the ground cinnamon and maple syrup (if using).
3. Divide the quinoa porridge into two bowls and top with chopped pecans and cranberries.
4. Serve warm.

TIPS:
- Add a dollop of lactose-free yogurt for extra creaminess.
- Substitute pecans with almonds or walnuts for variety.

N.V.: Calories: 320, Fat: 14g, Carbs: 42g, Protein: 8g, Sugar: 15g, Sodium: 30mg, Potassium: 300mg, Cholesterol: 0mg

TROPICAL QUINOA BREAKFAST BOWL

PREPARATION TIME: 5 min
COOKING TIME: 15 min
MODE OF COOKING: Stovetop
SERVINGS: 2
INGREDIENTS:

- 1/2 cup quinoa, rinsed
- 1 cup coconut milk (ensure it's low-FODMAP)
- 1/2 cup diced pineapple (fresh or frozen)
- 1/2 banana, sliced
- 2 Tbsp unsweetened shredded coconut
- 1 Tbsp chia seeds (optional)
- 1 Tbsp maple syrup (optional)

DIRECTIONS:

1. In a small saucepan, bring the coconut milk to a boil. Add the rinsed quinoa, reduce heat to low, cover, and simmer for 15 min or until the quinoa is tender and the liquid is absorbed.
2. Stir in the diced pineapple and sliced banana.
3. Divide the quinoa mixture into two bowls. Top with shredded coconut and chia seeds if using.
4. Drizzle with maple syrup if desired and serve warm.

TIPS:

- Add a sprinkle of cinnamon for extra warmth.
- Substitute pineapple with mango or papaya for variety.

N.V.: Calories: 350, Fat: 16g, Carbs: 45g, Protein: 8g, Sugar: 18g, Sodium: 50mg, Potassium: 400mg, Cholesterol: 0mg

STRAWBERRY AND ALMOND BUTTER OATMEAL BOWL

PREPARATION TIME: 5 min
COOKING TIME: 10 min
MODE OF COOKING: Stovetop
SERVINGS: 2
INGREDIENTS:

- 1 cup gluten-free rolled oats
- 2 cups lactose-free milk or water
- 1/2 cup fresh strawberries, sliced
- 2 Tbsp almond butter (ensure it's low-FODMAP)
- 1 Tbsp maple syrup (optional)
- 1/4 tsp ground cinnamon

DIRECTIONS:

1. In a medium saucepan, bring the lactose-free milk or water to a boil. Stir in the gluten-free rolled oats and reduce heat to low. Simmer for 5-7 min, stirring occasionally.
2. Stir in the almond butter, ground cinnamon, and maple syrup if using.
3. Divide the oatmeal into two bowls. Top with sliced strawberries.
4. Serve warm.

TIPS:

- Add a sprinkle of chia seeds for extra texture.
- Substitute strawberries with blueberries or raspberries for a different flavor.

N.V.: Calories: 320, Fat: 14g, Carbs: 42g, Protein: 10g, Sugar: 12g, Sodium: 30mg, Potassium: 350mg, Cholesterol: 0mg 4.3 Cozy and Warming Morning Meals

HEARTY PUMPKIN SPICE PANCAKES

PREPARATION TIME: 10 min
COOKING TIME: 15 min
MODE OF COOKING: Stovetop
SERVINGS: 4
INGREDIENTS:

- 1 cup gluten-free flour blend
- 1/2 cup canned pumpkin puree
- 1/2 cup lactose-free milk
- 2 large eggs
- 2 Tbsp maple syrup
- 1 tsp baking powder
- 1/2 tsp baking soda
- 1 tsp cinnamon
- 1/2 tsp ground ginger
- 1/4 tsp nutmeg
- 1/4 tsp salt
- 2 Tbsp melted coconut oil

DIRECTIONS:

1. In a large bowl, whisk together gluten-free flour, baking powder, baking soda, cinnamon, ginger, nutmeg, and salt.
2. In another bowl, mix together pumpkin puree, lactose-free milk, eggs, maple syrup, and melted coconut oil.
3. Pour the wet ingredients into the dry ingredients and stir until just combined.
4. Heat a non-stick skillet or griddle over medium heat and lightly grease with additional coconut oil.
5. Pour 1/4 cup of batter onto the skillet for each pancake. Cook until bubbles form on the surface, then flip and cook until golden brown.
6. Serve warm with a drizzle of maple syrup.

TIPS:

- Add a handful of chocolate chips to the batter for a sweet treat.
- Top with toasted pecans or walnuts for added crunch.

N.V.: Calories: 290, Fat: 12g, Carbs: 39g, Protein: 7g, Sugar: 10g, Sodium: 290mg, Potassium: 250mg, Cholesterol: 55mg

CREAMY COCONUT RICE PUDDING

PREPARATION TIME: 5 min
COOKING TIME: 20 min
MODE OF COOKING: Stovetop
SERVINGS: 4
INGREDIENTS:

- 1/2 cup jasmine rice
- 1 1/2 cups coconut milk
- 1/2 cup water
- 2 Tbsp maple syrup
- 1 tsp vanilla extract
- 1/4 tsp ground cinnamon
- Pinch of salt
- Fresh berries or chopped nuts for topping (optional)

DIRECTIONS:

1. In a medium saucepan, combine jasmine rice, coconut milk, water, maple syrup, vanilla extract, cinnamon, and salt.
2. Bring the mixture to a boil, then reduce the heat to low and cover.
3. Simmer for 20 min, stirring occasionally, until the rice is tender and the pudding is creamy.
4. Remove from heat and let sit for a few minutes before serving.
5. Serve warm, topped with fresh berries or chopped nuts if desired.

TIPS:

- For added flavor, stir in a spoonful of almond butter before serving.
- Store leftovers in the refrigerator and enjoy cold or reheated.

N.V.: Calories: 280, Fat: 12g, Carbs: 39g, Protein: 4g, Sugar: 10g, Sodium: 45mg, Potassium: 250mg, Cholesterol: 0mg

COZY VANILLA CHAI LATTE OATMEAL

PREPARATION TIME: 5 min
COOKING TIME: 10 min
MODE OF COOKING: Stovetop
SERVINGS: 2
INGREDIENTS:

- 1/2 cup gluten-free rolled oats
- 1 cup brewed chai tea (decaf if preferred)
- 1/2 cup lactose-free milk
- 1 Tbsp maple syrup
- 1/2 tsp vanilla extract
- Pinch of ground cinnamon
- 1 Tbsp almond butter (optional)

DIRECTIONS:

1. In a small saucepan, combine brewed chai tea, lactose-free milk, and oats.
2. Bring to a gentle boil over medium heat, then reduce the heat and simmer, stirring frequently, until the oats are tender and the mixture is creamy, about 10 min.

3. Stir in maple syrup, vanilla extract, and a pinch of cinnamon.
4. Divide oatmeal between two bowls and top with a swirl of almond butter if using. Serve warm.

TIPS:
- For extra richness, use coconut milk instead of lactose-free milk.
- Sprinkle with extra cinnamon on top for a warming finish.

N.V.: Calories: 220, Fat: 7g, Carbs: 35g, Protein: 5g, Sugar: 10g, Sodium: 55mg, Potassium: 250mg, Cholesterol: 0mg

WARM BANANA AND CINNAMON QUINOA

PREPARATION TIME: 5 min
COOKING TIME: 15 min
MODE OF COOKING: Stovetop
SERVINGS: 2
INGREDIENTS:
- 1/2 cup quinoa, rinsed
- 1 cup lactose-free milk or water
- 1 ripe banana, sliced
- 1/2 tsp ground cinnamon
- 1 Tbsp maple syrup (optional)
- 2 Tbsp chopped walnuts
- 1/4 tsp vanilla extract

DIRECTIONS:
1. In a small saucepan, bring the lactose-free milk or water to a boil. Add the rinsed quinoa, reduce heat, cover, and simmer for 15 min or until the quinoa is tender and the liquid is absorbed.
2. Stir in the sliced banana, ground cinnamon, vanilla extract, and maple syrup if using. Cook for an additional 2 min, stirring gently.
3. Divide the quinoa into two bowls and top with chopped walnuts.
4. Serve warm.

TIPS:
- Add a dollop of lactose-free yogurt for extra creaminess.
- Sprinkle with a pinch of nutmeg for additional warmth.

N.V.: Calories: 320, Fat: 10g, Carbs: 52g, Protein: 7g, Sugar: 16g, Sodium: 30mg, Potassium: 450mg, Cholesterol: 0mg

CREAMY POLENTA WITH SAUTÉED SPINACH AND EGG

PREPARATION TIME: 5 min
COOKING TIME: 15 min
MODE OF COOKING: Stovetop
SERVINGS: 2
INGREDIENTS:
- 1/2 cup polenta (cornmeal)
- 2 cups water or lactose-free milk
- 1 Tbsp lactose-free butter
- 1/4 cup lactose-free Parmesan cheese, grated
- 1 Tbsp olive oil
- 2 cups fresh spinach, chopped
- 2 large eggs
- Salt and pepper to taste
- 1/4 tsp smoked paprika (optional)

DIRECTIONS:
1. In a medium saucepan, bring the water or lactose-free milk to a boil. Gradually whisk in the polenta and reduce heat to low. Cook, stirring constantly, for 10 min or until thickened.
2. Stir in the lactose-free butter and grated Parmesan cheese. Season with salt and pepper to taste.
3. While the polenta is cooking, heat olive oil in a non-stick skillet over medium heat. Add the chopped spinach and sauté until wilted, about 3 min. Remove and set aside.
4. In the same skillet, fry the eggs to your desired doneness.
5. Divide the polenta into two bowls. Top with sautéed spinach and a fried egg. Sprinkle with smoked paprika if using.
6. Serve warm.

TIPS:
- Add a sprinkle of red pepper flakes for a spicy kick.

- Substitute spinach with kale or Swiss chard for variety.

N.V.: Calories: 350, Fat: 18g, Carbs: 34g, Protein: 14g, Sugar: 3g, Sodium: 250mg, Potassium: 550mg, Cholesterol: 210mg

BAKED PUMPKIN OATMEAL

PREPARATION TIME: 10 min
COOKING TIME: 20 min
MODE OF COOKING: Baking
SERVINGS: 4
INGREDIENTS:

- 2 cups gluten-free rolled oats
- 1 cup canned pumpkin puree (ensure it's low-FODMAP)
- 2 cups lactose-free milk
- 2 Tbsp maple syrup
- 1 tsp ground cinnamon
- 1/4 tsp ground nutmeg
- 1/4 tsp ground ginger
- 1 tsp vanilla extract
- 1/4 cup chopped pecans

DIRECTIONS:

1. Preheat oven to 375°F (190°C).
2. In a large mixing bowl, combine the gluten-free rolled oats, pumpkin puree, lactose-free milk, maple syrup, ground cinnamon, nutmeg, ginger, and vanilla extract. Mix until well combined.
3. Pour the mixture into a greased baking dish and spread evenly.
4. Sprinkle the top with chopped pecans.
5. Bake for 20 min, or until the oatmeal is set and slightly golden on top.
6. Serve warm, either on its own or with a drizzle of lactose-free milk.

TIPS:

- Add a handful of raisins or dried cranberries for extra sweetness.
- Serve with a dollop of lactose-free Greek yogurt for added protein.

N.V.: Calories: 280, Fat: 10g, Carbs: 42g, Protein: 6g, Sugar: 12g, Sodium: 50mg, Potassium: 400mg, Cholesterol: 0mg

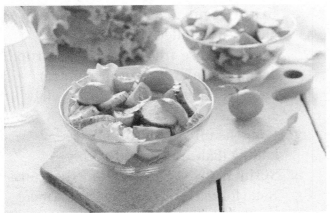

Navigating lunchtime can pose a unique challenge, especially for those of us on a low-FODMAP diet. It's an important opportunity to refuel midway through our day not just with calories, but with nutrition that suits our digestive needs without reintroducing symptoms we're all too eager to avoid. Imagine sitting down with a meal that nourishes and satisfies, that doesn't send you searching for symptoms or leave you feeling deprived. That's our goal for this chapter.

Life gets busy. Often, lunch is eaten hurriedly at a desk, in a school cafeteria, or even in the car. In these scenarios, the low-FODMAP diet might feel like a serious constraint. But it doesn't have to be. I've crafted a collection of recipes that cater to your life's pace while keeping flavor and variety at the forefront. Think of these dishes as quick culinary escapes during your busy day easy to prepare,

delightful to eat, and most importantly, safe for your gut.

From vibrant soups that can be whisked together the night before and warmed up at a moment's notice, to filling sandwiches made with low-FODMAP breads and fresh, crisp veggies that won't cause discomfort or bloating. And for those who need something even quicker, our quick lunch ideas will prove indispensable. These are meals that come together in a flash but feel gourmet.

We all want to enjoy our meals, not fear them. This chapter is about transforming lunchtime into a moment you look forward to, with meals that drive away monotony and bring in joy and comfort without forsaking your dietary needs. Whether you're cooking for one at home or packing up your lunchbox for work, these recipes are designed to fit seamlessly into your day and provide the kind of midday pause that becomes a cherished part of your routine.

Embrace these recipes as your toolkit for turning a meal often eaten on autopilot into something truly special and beneficial for your digestive health. Let's make every lunch nourishing and no-fuss, with flavors that excite and satisfy every palate, including yours.

QUINOA AND KALE SALAD WITH LEMON VINAIGRETTE

PREPARATION TIME: 15 min
COOKING TIME: 15 min
MODE OF COOKING: Stovetop
SERVINGS: 4
INGREDIENTS:

- 1 cup quinoa, rinsed
- 2 cups water
- 4 cups kale, chopped (stems removed)
- 1/2 cup cherry tomatoes, halved
- 1/4 cup sliced almonds, toasted
- 1/4 cup crumbled feta cheese (optional)

Lemon Vinaigrette:

- 1/4 cup olive oil
- 2 Tbsp fresh lemon juice
- 1 tsp Dijon mustard
- 1 tsp maple syrup
- Salt and pepper to taste

DIRECTIONS:

1. In a medium saucepan, bring water to a boil. Add quinoa, reduce heat, cover, and simmer for 15 min or until water is absorbed.
2. While quinoa cooks, prepare the vinaigrette by whisking together olive oil, lemon juice, Dijon mustard, maple syrup, salt, and pepper in a small bowl.
3. In a large bowl, combine chopped kale, cherry tomatoes, and cooked quinoa.
4. Pour the vinaigrette over the salad and toss well to coat.
5. Sprinkle with toasted almonds and crumbled feta cheese if using. Serve immediately.

TIPS:

- Massage the kale with a little olive oil before mixing for a softer texture.
- Add grilled chicken or tofu for extra protein.

N.V.: Calories: 280, Fat: 15g, Carbs: 30g, Protein: 8g, Sugar: 4g, Sodium: 120mg, Potassium: 550mg, Cholesterol: 0mg

AVOCADO AND CITRUS SALAD

PREPARATION TIME: 10 min
COOKING TIME: 0 min
MODE OF COOKING: No Cooking
SERVINGS: 4
INGREDIENTS:

- 2 ripe avocados, sliced
- 2 oranges, peeled and segmented
- 1 grapefruit, peeled and segmented
- 1/4 cup red onion, thinly sliced (green parts only for low-FODMAP)
- 1/4 cup fresh mint leaves, chopped
- 2 Tbsp olive oil
- 1 Tbsp fresh lime juice
- Salt and pepper to taste

DIRECTIONS:

1. In a large bowl, combine sliced avocados, orange segments, grapefruit segments, and red onion.
2. In a small bowl, whisk together olive oil, lime juice, salt, and pepper.
3. Pour the dressing over the salad and toss gently to combine.
4. Garnish with fresh mint leaves and serve immediately.

TIPS:

- Add a handful of arugula or baby spinach for added greens.
- Top with toasted pumpkin seeds for a crunchy texture.

N.V.: Calories: 220, Fat: 17g, Carbs: 18g, Protein: 2g, Sugar: 9g, Sodium: 10mg, Potassium: 600mg, Cholesterol: 0mg

ZUCCHINI AND LEMON SOUP

PREPARATION TIME: 10 min
COOKING TIME: 20 min
MODE OF COOKING: Stovetop
SERVINGS: 4
INGREDIENTS:

- 4 small zucchinis, chopped
- 1 Tbsp olive oil

- 1/2 tsp dried thyme
- 3 cups low-sodium vegetable broth
- 1/2 cup lactose-free Greek yogurt
- 1 lemon, juiced and zested
- Salt and pepper to taste
- Fresh dill for garnish

DIRECTIONS:

1. In a large pot, heat the olive oil over medium heat. Add the chopped zucchini and dried thyme. Sauté for 5-7 min, or until the zucchini is tender.
2. Pour in the vegetable broth and bring to a boil. Reduce heat and simmer for 10 min.
3. Remove from heat and blend the soup until smooth using an immersion blender or a regular blender.
4. Stir in the lactose-free Greek yogurt, lemon juice, and lemon zest. Season with salt and pepper to taste.
5. Serve hot, garnished with fresh dill.

TIPS:

- Add a handful of spinach during the last 2 minutes of cooking for added nutrients.
- Serve with a side of gluten-free crackers or bread.

N.V.: Calories: 130, Fat: 7g, Carbs: 14g, Protein: 5g, Sugar: 6g, Sodium: 320mg, Potassium: 500mg, Cholesterol: 5mg

SIMPLE TOMATO AND CUCUMBER SALAD

PREPARATION TIME: 10 min
COOKING TIME: 0 min
MODE OF COOKING: No Cooking
SERVINGS: 4
INGREDIENTS:

- 2 large tomatoes, diced
- 1 cucumber, peeled and diced
- 1/4 cup lactose-free feta cheese, crumbled
- 2 Tbsp olive oil
- 1 Tbsp balsamic vinegar
- 1/2 tsp dried oregano
- Salt and pepper to taste

- Fresh basil leaves for garnish

DIRECTIONS:

1. In a large bowl, combine the diced tomatoes, cucumber, and crumbled lactose-free feta cheese.
2. In a small bowl, whisk together the olive oil, balsamic vinegar, dried oregano, salt, and pepper.
3. Pour the dressing over the salad and toss gently to combine.
4. Garnish with fresh basil leaves and serve immediately.

TIPS:

- Add a handful of olives for extra flavor.
- Serve as a side dish with grilled chicken or fish.

N.V.: Calories: 120, Fat: 10g, Carbs: 8g, Protein: 3g, Sugar: 4g, Sodium: 150mg, Potassium: 350mg, Cholesterol: 5mg

SPINACH AND STRAWBERRY SALAD WITH LEMON VINAIGRETTE

PREPARATION TIME: 10 min
COOKING TIME: 0 min
MODE OF COOKING: No Cooking
SERVINGS: 4
INGREDIENTS:

- 4 cups fresh spinach, washed and dried
- 1 cup fresh strawberries, sliced
- 1/4 cup chopped walnuts
- 1/4 cup lactose-free feta cheese, crumbled (optional)
- 2 Tbsp olive oil
- 1 Tbsp lemon juice
- 1 tsp Dijon mustard
- Salt and pepper to taste

DIRECTIONS:

1. In a large bowl, combine the fresh spinach, sliced strawberries, chopped walnuts, and crumbled lactose-free feta cheese.
2. In a small bowl, whisk together the olive oil, lemon juice, Dijon mustard, salt, and pepper.

3. Pour the lemon vinaigrette over the salad and toss gently to coat.
4. Serve immediately.

TIPS:
- Add grilled chicken or shrimp for a heartier salad.
- Substitute walnuts with pecans or almonds for variety.

N.V.: Calories: 180, Fat: 14g, Carbs: 10g, Protein: 4g, Sugar: 4g, Sodium: 120mg, Potassium: 350mg, Cholesterol: 5mg

WARM QUINOA AND ROASTED VEGETABLE SALAD

PREPARATION TIME: 10 min
COOKING TIME: 20 min
MODE OF COOKING: Roasting and Stovetop
SERVINGS: 4
INGREDIENTS:
- 1 cup quinoa, rinsed
- 2 cups water or low-sodium vegetable broth
- 1 zucchini, diced
- 1 red bell pepper, diced
- 1 carrot, peeled and diced
- 2 Tbsp olive oil
- 1/2 tsp dried thyme
- Salt and pepper to taste
- 1/4 cup lactose-free feta cheese, crumbled (optional)
- Fresh parsley for garnish

DIRECTIONS:
1. Preheat the oven to 400°F (204°C).
2. Toss the diced zucchini, red bell pepper, and carrot with olive oil, dried thyme, salt, and pepper. Spread the vegetables on a baking sheet and roast for 20 min, or until tender.
3. While the vegetables are roasting, cook the quinoa by bringing water or vegetable broth to a boil in a medium saucepan. Add the quinoa, reduce heat, cover, and simmer for 15 min, or until the quinoa is tender and the liquid is absorbed.

4. Fluff the quinoa with a fork and transfer to a large bowl. Add the roasted vegetables and toss to combine.
5. Sprinkle with crumbled lactose-free feta cheese and garnish with fresh parsley before serving.

TIPS:
- Add a handful of spinach or arugula for extra greens.
- Serve warm or at room temperature.

N.V.: Calories: 250, Fat: 10g, Carbs: 32g, Protein: 6g, Sugar: 6g, Sodium: 220mg, Potassium: 500mg, Cholesterol: 5mg

GRILLED CHICKEN AVOCADO WRAP

PREPARATION TIME: 10 min
COOKING TIME: 10 min
MODE OF COOKING: Grilling
SERVINGS: 2
INGREDIENTS:
- 2 small boneless, skinless chicken breasts
- 1 Tbsp olive oil
- 1/2 tsp paprika
- Salt and pepper to taste
- 2 gluten-free wraps
- 1 ripe avocado, sliced
- 1/2 cup baby spinach
- 1/4 cup lactose-free Greek yogurt
- 1 Tbsp fresh lemon juice

DIRECTIONS:
1. Preheat the grill to medium-high heat.
2. Rub the chicken breasts with olive oil, paprika, salt, and pepper.
3. Grill the chicken for 5-7 min per side, or until fully cooked. Let it rest for a few minutes, then slice thinly.
4. In a small bowl, mix lactose-free Greek yogurt with fresh lemon juice.
5. Lay the gluten-free wraps on a flat surface. Spread the yogurt mixture on each wrap.
6. Layer the sliced chicken, avocado, and baby spinach on the wraps.

7. Roll up the wraps tightly and slice in half to serve.

TIPS:
- Add a slice of tomato for extra freshness.
- Use a panini press to toast the wrap for added crunch.

N.V.: Calories: 390, Fat: 20g, Carbs: 25g, Protein: 30g, Sugar: 2g, Sodium: 360mg, Potassium: 700mg, Cholesterol: 75mg

TURKEY AND SWISS LETTUCE WRAPS

PREPARATION TIME: 10 min
COOKING TIME: 0 min
MODE OF COOKING: No Cooking
SERVINGS: 2
INGREDIENTS:
- 4 large romaine lettuce leaves
- 6 slices deli turkey (nitrate-free)
- 2 slices Swiss cheese (lactose-free)
- 1/2 avocado, sliced
- 1/4 cup shredded carrots
- 1 Tbsp Dijon mustard
- Salt and pepper to taste

DIRECTIONS:
1. Lay the lettuce leaves on a flat surface.
2. Spread a thin layer of Dijon mustard on each lettuce leaf.
3. Layer 3 slices of turkey, 1 slice of Swiss cheese, avocado slices, and shredded carrots on each leaf.
4. Season with salt and pepper.
5. Roll up the lettuce leaves tightly, securing with toothpicks if needed. Serve immediately.

TIPS:
- Substitute Swiss cheese with lactose-free cheddar for a different flavor.
- Add a slice of red bell pepper for a sweet crunch.

N.V.: Calories: 220, Fat: 14g, Carbs: 6g, Protein: 18g, Sugar: 2g, Sodium: 450mg, Potassium: 420mg, Cholesterol: 50mg

MEDITERRANEAN VEGGIE PITA SANDWICH

PREPARATION TIME: 10 min
COOKING TIME: 5 min
MODE OF COOKING: Stovetop
SERVINGS: 2
INGREDIENTS:
- 2 gluten-free pita pockets
- 1/2 cup hummus (low-FODMAP)
- 1/4 cup cucumber, diced
- 1/4 cup cherry tomatoes, halved
- 1/4 cup Kalamata olives, sliced
- 1/4 cup feta cheese, crumbled (lactose-free)
- 1/4 cup baby spinach
- 1 Tbsp fresh parsley, chopped

DIRECTIONS:
1. Warm the pita pockets on a stovetop or in a toaster.
2. Cut the pitas in half and carefully open each half to form a pocket.
3. Spread hummus inside each pita pocket.
4. Stuff the pita with cucumber, cherry tomatoes, olives, feta cheese, and baby spinach.
5. Sprinkle with fresh parsley and serve.

TIPS:
- Add a squeeze of fresh lemon juice for extra zest.
- Substitute hummus with lactose-free tzatziki for a refreshing twist.

N.V.: Calories: 340, Fat: 16g, Carbs: 38g, Protein: 12g, Sugar: 4g, Sodium: 620mg, Potassium: 350mg, Cholesterol: 15mg

TUNA SALAD COLLARD WRAPS

PREPARATION TIME: 10 min
COOKING TIME: 0 min
MODE OF COOKING: No Cooking
SERVINGS: 2
INGREDIENTS:
- 1 can (5 oz) tuna in water, drained
- 2 Tbsp lactose-free mayonnaise
- 1 Tbsp fresh lemon juice

- 1 Tbsp fresh dill, chopped
- Salt and pepper to taste
- 4 large collard green leaves
- 1/2 avocado, sliced
- 1/4 cup shredded carrots

DIRECTIONS:

1. In a bowl, mix together the drained tuna, lactose-free mayonnaise, lemon juice, dill, salt, and pepper.
2. Lay the collard green leaves on a flat surface.
3. Divide the tuna salad evenly among the leaves.
4. Top with avocado slices and shredded carrots.
5. Roll up the collard greens like a burrito, folding in the sides as you go. Serve immediately.

TIPS:

- Add a dash of hot sauce to the tuna salad for a spicy kick.
- Use lettuce leaves instead of collard greens for a milder flavor.

N.V.: Calories: 270, Fat: 17g, Carbs: 10g, Protein: 22g, Sugar: 2g, Sodium: 330mg, Potassium: 550mg, Cholesterol: 40mg

GRILLED VEGGIE AND HUMMUS WRAP

PREPARATION TIME: 15 min
COOKING TIME: 10 min
MODE OF COOKING: Grilling
SERVINGS: 2
INGREDIENTS:

- 1 zucchini, sliced lengthwise
- 1 red bell pepper, sliced into strips
- 1 yellow bell pepper, sliced into strips
- 1 Tbsp olive oil
- Salt and pepper to taste
- 2 gluten-free wraps
- 1/2 cup hummus (low-FODMAP)
- 1/4 cup crumbled feta cheese (lactose-free)
- 1/4 cup fresh basil leaves

DIRECTIONS:

1. Preheat the grill to medium-high heat.

2. Toss the zucchini and bell pepper slices with olive oil, salt, and pepper.
3. Grill the vegetables for 3-4 min per side, until tender and slightly charred.
4. Spread hummus on each gluten-free wrap.
5. Layer the grilled vegetables on top of the hummus.
6. Sprinkle with crumbled feta cheese and fresh basil leaves.
7. Roll up the wraps and slice in half to serve.

TIPS:

- Add a drizzle of balsamic glaze for extra flavor.
- Use a mix of different colored bell peppers for a vibrant presentation.

N.V.: Calories: 310, Fat: 16g, Carbs: 33g, Protein: 8g, Sugar: 8g, Sodium: 380mg, Potassium: 450mg, Cholesterol: 15mg

SPICY CHICKEN SALAD WRAP

PREPARATION TIME: 10 min
COOKING TIME: 10 min
MODE OF COOKING: Stovetop
SERVINGS: 2
INGREDIENTS:

- 2 small boneless, skinless chicken breasts
- 1 Tbsp olive oil
- 1 tsp smoked paprika
- 1/2 tsp cumin
- Salt and pepper to taste
- 2 gluten-free wraps
- 1/4 cup lactose-free Greek yogurt
- 1 Tbsp fresh lime juice
- 1/2 avocado, sliced
- 1/4 cup shredded lettuce
- 1/4 cup chopped cilantro

DIRECTIONS:

1. Heat olive oil in a skillet over medium heat.
2. Season the chicken breasts with smoked paprika, cumin, salt, and pepper.

3. Cook the chicken in the skillet for 5-7 min per side, or until fully cooked. Let it rest for a few minutes, then slice thinly.
4. In a small bowl, mix lactose-free Greek yogurt with fresh lime juice.
5. Spread the yogurt mixture on the gluten-free wraps.
6. Layer the sliced chicken, avocado, shredded lettuce, and chopped cilantro on the wraps.
7. Roll up the wraps and slice in half to serve.

TIPS:
- Add a few jalapeño slices for an extra spicy kick.
- Serve with a side of salsa for dipping.

N.V.: Calories: 380, Fat: 18g, Carbs: 25g, Protein: 30g, Sugar: 2g, Sodium: 370mg, Potassium: 700mg, Cholesterol: 75mg

CAPRESE SALAD WITH QUINOA

PREPARATION TIME: 10 min
COOKING TIME: 15 min
MODE OF COOKING: Stovetop
SERVINGS: 2
INGREDIENTS:
- 1/2 cup quinoa, rinsed
- 1 cup water
- 1 cup cherry tomatoes, halved
- 1/4 cup fresh mozzarella balls (lactose-free), halved
- 1/4 cup fresh basil leaves, chopped
- 2 Tbsp balsamic vinegar
- 1 Tbsp olive oil
- Salt and pepper to taste

DIRECTIONS:
1. In a small saucepan, combine quinoa and water. Bring to a boil, then reduce heat, cover, and simmer for 15 min, or until water is absorbed.
2. Fluff the quinoa with a fork and let it cool slightly.
3. In a large bowl, combine the cooked quinoa, cherry tomatoes, mozzarella, and fresh basil.

4. Drizzle with balsamic vinegar and olive oil, then toss to combine.
5. Season with salt and pepper to taste. Serve immediately.

TIPS:
- Add a handful of arugula for extra greens.
- Use gluten-free croutons for added crunch.

N.V.: Calories: 320, Fat: 16g, Carbs: 32g, Protein: 10g, Sugar: 5g, Sodium: 120mg, Potassium: 450mg, Cholesterol: 10mg

AVOCADO TOAST WITH POACHED EGG

PREPARATION TIME: 5 min
COOKING TIME: 5 min
MODE OF COOKING: Stovetop
SERVINGS: 2
INGREDIENTS:
- 2 slices gluten-free bread, toasted
- 1 ripe avocado, mashed
- 2 large eggs
- 1 tsp vinegar
- Salt and pepper to taste
- Red pepper flakes (optional)

DIRECTIONS:
1. Bring a pot of water to a gentle simmer. Add vinegar to the water.
2. Crack the eggs into separate small bowls. Create a gentle whirlpool in the water, then gently slide each egg into the water. Poach for 3-4 min until whites are set and yolks are runny.
3. While the eggs are poaching, spread mashed avocado onto the toasted gluten-free bread slices.
4. Carefully remove the poached eggs from the water using a slotted spoon, and place one on each slice of avocado toast.
5. Season with salt, pepper, and red pepper flakes if using. Serve immediately.

TIPS:
- Add a squeeze of fresh lemon juice to the avocado for extra flavor.

- Top with cherry tomatoes or radish slices for a colorful garnish.

N.V.: Calories: 300, Fat: 20g, Carbs: 20g, Protein: 12g, Sugar: 2g, Sodium: 200mg, Potassium: 550mg, Cholesterol: 185mg

VEGGIE-PACKED HUMMUS WRAP

PREPARATION TIME: 10 min
COOKING TIME: 0 min
MODE OF COOKING: No Cooking
SERVINGS: 2
INGREDIENTS:

- 2 gluten-free wraps
- 1/2 cup hummus (low-FODMAP)
- 1/4 cup cucumber, julienned
- 1/4 cup red bell pepper, julienned
- 1/4 cup shredded carrots
- 1/4 cup baby spinach
- 1 Tbsp fresh parsley, chopped
- 1 Tbsp fresh lemon juice
- Salt and pepper to taste

DIRECTIONS:

1. Lay the gluten-free wraps on a flat surface.
2. Spread hummus evenly over each wrap.
3. Layer cucumber, red bell pepper, shredded carrots, baby spinach, and fresh parsley on top of the hummus.
4. Drizzle with fresh lemon juice and season with salt and pepper.
5. Roll up the wraps tightly, slice in half, and serve.

TIPS:

- Add a slice of avocado for extra creaminess.
- Serve with a side of mixed greens for a complete meal.

N.V.: Calories: 310, Fat: 12g, Carbs: 42g, Protein: 8g, Sugar: 6g, Sodium: 320mg, Potassium: 450mg, Cholesterol: 0mg

SHRIMP AND AVOCADO SALAD

PREPARATION TIME: 10 min
COOKING TIME: 5 min
MODE OF COOKING: Stovetop
SERVINGS: 2
INGREDIENTS:

- 1/2 lb. shrimp, peeled and deveined
- 1 Tbsp olive oil
- 1 avocado, diced
- 1 cup cherry tomatoes, halved
- 1/4 cup red onion, thinly sliced (green parts only for low-FODMAP)
- 2 Tbsp fresh cilantro, chopped
- 1 Tbsp fresh lime juice
- Salt and pepper to taste

DIRECTIONS:

1. Heat olive oil in a skillet over medium heat.
2. Add shrimp to the skillet and cook for 2-3 min per side, until opaque and cooked through. Remove from heat and let cool slightly.
3. In a large bowl, combine diced avocado, cherry tomatoes, red onion, and cooked shrimp.
4. Drizzle with fresh lime juice, and toss to combine.
5. Season with salt, pepper, and fresh cilantro. Serve immediately.

TIPS:

- Add a pinch of cayenne pepper for a spicy kick.
- Serve over a bed of mixed greens for a more substantial meal.

N.V.: Calories: 280, Fat: 18g, Carbs: 12g, Protein: 20g, Sugar: 3g, Sodium: 300mg, Potassium: 650mg, Cholesterol: 140mg

QUICK TUNA SALAD WITH CUCUMBER

PREPARATION TIME: 10 min
COOKING TIME: 0 min
MODE OF COOKING: No Cooking
SERVINGS: 2
INGREDIENTS:

- 1 can (5 oz) tuna in water, drained
- 1/2 cucumber, diced
- 1/4 cup lactose-free Greek yogurt
- 1 Tbsp Dijon mustard
- 1 Tbsp lemon juice
- 1 Tbsp chopped fresh dill (optional)
- Salt and pepper to taste
- Lettuce leaves for serving

DIRECTIONS:

1. In a medium bowl, combine the drained tuna, diced cucumber, lactose-free Greek yogurt, Dijon mustard, lemon juice, and chopped dill if using.
2. Mix well until all ingredients are evenly distributed. Season with salt and pepper to taste.
3. Serve the tuna salad in lettuce leaves for a light and refreshing lunch.

TIPS:

- Add a hard-boiled egg for extra protein.
- Serve with gluten-free crackers or toast for added crunch.

N.V.: Calories: 180, Fat: 6g, Carbs: 8g, Protein: 24g, Sugar: 2g, Sodium: 300mg, Potassium: 350mg, Cholesterol: 40mg

CHICKEN AND AVOCADO WRAP

PREPARATION TIME: 10 min
COOKING TIME: 0 min
MODE OF COOKING: No Cooking
SERVINGS: 2
INGREDIENTS:

- 2 gluten-free tortillas
- 1 cup cooked chicken breast, shredded
- 1 ripe avocado, sliced
- 1/2 cup lactose-free Greek yogurt
- 1/4 cup grated lactose-free cheddar cheese
- 1/2 cup fresh spinach leaves
- 1/4 tsp smoked paprika
- Salt and pepper to taste

DIRECTIONS:

1. In a small bowl, mix the shredded chicken with the lactose-free Greek yogurt, smoked paprika, salt, and pepper.
2. Lay out the gluten-free tortillas and divide the chicken mixture evenly between them.
3. Top each tortilla with sliced avocado, grated cheese, and fresh spinach leaves.
4. Roll up the tortillas tightly and slice them in half.
5. Serve immediately.

TIPS:

- Add a squeeze of lime juice to the avocado for extra freshness.
- Substitute the chicken with turkey or ham for variety.

N.V.: Calories: 360, Fat: 20g, Carbs: 26g, Protein: 22g, Sugar: 2g, Sodium: 300mg, Potassium: 650mg, Cholesterol: 60mg

CHAPTER 7: DINNER INSPIRATIONS

As the day winds down and evening sets in, the kitchen becomes not just a place for meal preparation, but a sanctuary where flavors blend and simmer to create comforting dinners that wrap up our day. In this chapter, you'll discover dinner options that promise not just to nourish but to delight, crafting moments of joy for you and your loved ones, regardless of your dietary restrictions.

Think of a warm kitchen filled with the inviting aromas of a simmering pot this is where the low-FODMAP diet transforms from a dietary requirement to an opportunity for culinary creativity. Here, traditional family favorites are reimagined to suit your needs without compromising taste or satisfaction. Whether you're gathered around the table for a family dinner or enjoying a quiet meal by yourself, these recipes are designed to ensure that everyone at the table can indulge in the moment, appreciating both the delicious food and the company they share.

Imagine transforming a typical high-FODMAP meal into a gut-friendly feast. With a few simple ingredient swaps, a dish like lasagna, often laden with garlic and onions, becomes a soothing, safe haven that's just as rich and flavorful with a low-FODMAP garlic-infused oil or a sprinkle of chives for a gentle, onion-free kick. It's all about maintaining the depth of flavor while keeping your digestive comfort in mind.

Throughout this chapter, we'll explore a variety of dinners, from quick one-pot meals perfect for those busier evenings to more elaborate dishes that bring the whole family together. These aren't just recipes; they're your pathway to reclaiming the joy of cooking and eating, no matter the dietary restrictions. With each dish, you'll find practical tips to tweak and tailor recipes according to your current phase in the low-FODMAP diet, making it simpler to manage your symptoms while still enjoying a diverse and flavorful dinner menu.

This chapter is an invitation: to keep dinner interesting, healthful, and above all, delicious. So, tie on your apron, and let's make dinner a highlight of your day where good health and great flavors meet on your plate.

HERB-ROASTED CHICKEN WITH LEMON AND ROSEMARY

PREPARATION TIME: 10 min
COOKING TIME: 20 min
MODE OF COOKING: Oven Roasting
SERVINGS: 4
INGREDIENTS:

- 4 boneless, skinless chicken breasts
- 2 Tbsp olive oil
- 1 lemon, juiced and zested
- 1 Tbsp fresh rosemary, chopped
- 1 tsp dried thyme
- Salt and pepper to taste
- 1 tsp garlic-infused olive oil (optional, for added flavor)

DIRECTIONS:

1. Preheat oven to 400°F (204°C).
2. In a bowl, combine olive oil, lemon juice, zest, rosemary, thyme, salt, and pepper.
3. Rub the chicken breasts with the herb mixture.
4. Place the chicken on a baking sheet lined with parchment paper.
5. Roast in the oven for 20 minutes or until the chicken reaches an internal temperature of 165°F (74°C).
6. Let the chicken rest for 5 minutes before serving.

TIPS:

- Serve with a side of roasted potatoes and steamed spinach for a complete meal.
- Use the leftover lemon herb sauce for a light salad dressing.

N.V.: Calories: 220, Fat: 10g, Carbs: 2g, Protein: 28g, Sugar: 0g, Sodium: 75 mg, Potassium: 320 mg, Cholesterol: 75 mg

QUICK AND EASY BEEF STIR-FRY

PREPARATION TIME: 10 min
COOKING TIME: 10 min
MODE OF COOKING: Stir-Frying
SERVINGS: 4
INGREDIENTS:

- 1 lb. beef sirloin, thinly sliced
- 1 Tbsp olive oil
- 1 red bell pepper, sliced
- 1 zucchini, sliced
- 2 carrots, julienned
- 2 Tbsp tamari (gluten-free soy sauce)
- 1 Tbsp rice vinegar
- 1 tsp ginger, grated
- 1 tsp garlic-infused olive oil
- 1 tsp sesame oil (optional)

DIRECTIONS:

1. Heat olive oil in a large pan over medium-high heat.
2. Add beef slices and stir-fry until browned, about 3 minutes.
3. Add bell pepper, zucchini, and carrots to the pan and stir-fry for 5 minutes.
4. Stir in tamari, rice vinegar, ginger, and garlic-infused oil.
5. Cook for an additional 2 minutes, or until vegetables are tender-crisp.
6. Drizzle with sesame oil before serving, if using.

TIPS:

- Serve over a bed of rice or quinoa for a heartier meal.
- Garnish with chopped green onions for added freshness.

N.V.: Calories: 290, Fat: 15g, Carbs: 8g, Protein: 30g, Sugar: 4g, Sodium: 570 mg, Potassium: 550 mg, Cholesterol: 70 mg

BAKED SALMON WITH DILL AND CITRUS

PREPARATION TIME: 5 min
COOKING TIME: 20 min
MODE OF COOKING: Baking
SERVINGS: 4
INGREDIENTS:

- 4 salmon fillets
- 2 Tbsp olive oil
- 1 lemon, thinly sliced
- 1 Tbsp fresh dill, chopped
- Salt and pepper to taste

- 1 tsp garlic-infused olive oil (optional, for added flavor)

DIRECTIONS:

1. Preheat oven to 375°F (190°C).
2. Place salmon fillets on a baking sheet lined with parchment paper.
3. Drizzle olive oil and garlic-infused olive oil over the fillets.
4. Season with salt, pepper, and dill.
5. Lay lemon slices over each fillet.
6. Bake for 15-20 minutes, or until the salmon flakes easily with a fork.

TIPS:

- Serve with a side of quinoa and steamed green beans.
- Add a sprinkle of freshly chopped parsley for added color.

N.V.: Calories: 350, Fat: 20g, Carbs: 3g, Protein: 37g, Sugar: 0g, Sodium: 60 mg, Potassium: 450 mg, Cholesterol: 90 mg

ONE-POT CHICKEN AND RICE

PREPARATION TIME: 10 min
COOKING TIME: 20 min
MODE OF COOKING: Stovetop
SERVINGS: 4
INGREDIENTS:

- 4 boneless, skinless chicken thighs
- 1 cup white rice, rinsed
- 2 cups low-sodium chicken broth
- 1 carrot, diced
- 1 zucchini, diced
- 1 tsp dried thyme
- 1 Tbsp olive oil
- Salt and pepper to taste

DIRECTIONS:

1. Heat olive oil in a large pot over medium heat.
2. Add chicken thighs, seasoning with salt and pepper, and cook until browned on both sides, about 5 minutes.
3. Remove chicken and set aside.
4. Add rice, broth, carrot, zucchini, and thyme to the pot.

5. Stir well, then return the chicken to the pot, placing it on top of the rice.
6. Cover and simmer for 20 minutes, or until rice is cooked and chicken is tender.

TIPS:

- For added flavor, sprinkle with fresh parsley before serving.
- Substitute brown rice for a whole-grain option, increasing the cooking time by 10 minutes.

N.V.: Calories: 420, Fat: 15g, Carbs: 45g, Protein: 28g, Sugar: 2g, Sodium: 450 mg, Potassium: 400 mg, Cholesterol: 95 mg

EASY TURKEY MEATLOAF

PREPARATION TIME: 10 min
COOKING TIME: 20 min
MODE OF COOKING: Baking
SERVINGS: 4
INGREDIENTS:

- 1 lb. ground turkey
- 1/2 cup gluten-free breadcrumbs
- 1 egg
- 1 Tbsp tomato paste
- 1 tsp Worcestershire sauce
- 1 tsp dried oregano
- Salt and pepper to taste
- 1 Tbsp olive oil

DIRECTIONS:

1. Preheat oven to 375°F (190°C).
2. In a large bowl, combine ground turkey, breadcrumbs, egg, tomato paste, Worcestershire sauce, oregano, salt, and pepper.
3. Shape the mixture into a loaf and place it in a greased baking dish.
4. Drizzle with olive oil.
5. Bake for 20 minutes or until the internal temperature reaches 165°F (74°C).

TIPS:

- Serve with a side of mashed potatoes and steamed green beans.

- Add a small grated carrot to the meatloaf mixture for extra moisture and flavor.

N.V.: Calories: 280, Fat: 12g, Carbs: 12g, Protein: 30g, Sugar: 2g, Sodium: 320 mg, Potassium: 450 mg, Cholesterol: 120 mg

SHRIMP AND VEGETABLE SKEWERS

PREPARATION TIME: 10 min
COOKING TIME: 10 min
MODE OF COOKING: Grilling
SERVINGS: 4
INGREDIENTS:

- 1 lb. large shrimp, peeled and deveined
- 1 red bell pepper, cut into chunks
- 1 zucchini, sliced
- 1 yellow squash, sliced
- 2 Tbsp olive oil
- 1 tsp dried oregano
- 1 lemon, juiced
- Salt and pepper to taste
- Wooden or metal skewers

DIRECTIONS:

1. Preheat grill to medium-high heat.
2. In a bowl, toss shrimp and vegetables with olive oil, lemon juice, oregano, salt, and pepper.
3. Thread shrimp and vegetables onto skewers.
4. Grill skewers for 2-3 minutes per side, or until shrimp are opaque and vegetables are tender.

TIPS:

- Serve over a bed of quinoa or rice.
- For extra flavor, brush skewers with additional lemon juice before serving.

N.V.: Calories: 210, Fat: 9g, Carbs: 8g, Protein: 25g, Sugar: 3g, Sodium: 350 mg, Potassium: 450 mg, Cholesterol: 180 mg

ONE-POT SHRIMP AND VEGETABLE PASTA

PREPARATION TIME: 10 min
COOKING TIME: 20 min
MODE OF COOKING: Stovetop
SERVINGS: 4
INGREDIENTS:

- 1 lb. large shrimp, peeled and deveined
- 8 oz gluten-free pasta
- 2 cups low-sodium chicken broth
- 1 zucchini, diced
- 1 red bell pepper, diced
- 1 tsp dried basil
- 1 Tbsp olive oil
- 1 tsp garlic-infused olive oil
- Salt and pepper to taste
- Fresh basil for garnish

DIRECTIONS:

1. Heat olive oil in a large pot over medium heat.
2. Add shrimp and cook until pink, about 3 minutes. Remove and set aside.
3. Add pasta, chicken broth, zucchini, bell pepper, dried basil, and garlic-infused oil to the pot.
4. Bring to a boil, then reduce heat and simmer, uncovered, for 15 minutes or until pasta is al dente.
5. Return shrimp to the pot and cook for an additional 2 minutes, until heated through.
6. Garnish with fresh basil before serving.

TIPS:

- Serve with a side of garlic-infused olive oil bread for a complete meal.
- Add a pinch of red pepper flakes for a bit of heat.

N.V.: Calories: 360, Fat: 8g, Carbs: 40g, Protein: 30g, Sugar: 4g, Sodium: 430 mg, Potassium: 600 mg, Cholesterol: 180 mg

ONE-POT ITALIAN SAUSAGE AND RICE SKILLET

PREPARATION TIME: 10 min
COOKING TIME: 20 min
MODE OF COOKING: Stovetop
SERVINGS: 4
INGREDIENTS:

- 4 Italian sausage links (low-FODMAP, gluten-free)
- 1 cup white rice, rinsed
- 2 cups low-sodium chicken broth
- 1 red bell pepper, diced
- 1 zucchini, diced
- 1 tsp dried oregano
- 1 Tbsp olive oil
- Salt and pepper to taste

DIRECTIONS:

1. Heat olive oil in a large skillet over medium heat.
2. Cook the sausage links until browned on all sides, about 5 minutes.
3. Remove sausages from the skillet and set aside.
4. Add rice, chicken broth, bell pepper, zucchini, and oregano to the skillet. Stir to combine.
5. Return the sausages to the skillet, nestling them into the rice mixture.
6. Cover and simmer for 20 minutes or until rice is tender and sausages are cooked through.

TIPS:

- Add a sprinkle of grated lactose-free Parmesan cheese for extra flavor.
- Serve with a simple side salad for a balanced meal.

N.V.: Calories: 400, Fat: 20g, Carbs: 35g, Protein: 20g, Sugar: 4g, Sodium: 720 mg, Potassium: 450 mg, Cholesterol: 60 mg

ONE-POT LEMON GARLIC CHICKEN WITH QUINOA

PREPARATION TIME: 10 min
COOKING TIME: 20 min
MODE OF COOKING: Stovetop
SERVINGS: 4
INGREDIENTS:

- 4 boneless, skinless chicken thighs
- 1 cup quinoa, rinsed
- 2 cups low-sodium chicken broth
- 1 lemon, juiced and zested
- 1 Tbsp olive oil
- 1 tsp garlic-infused olive oil
- 1 zucchini, diced
- 1 red bell pepper, diced
- 1 tsp dried thyme
- Salt and pepper to taste

DIRECTIONS:

1. Heat olive oil in a large pot over medium heat.
2. Season chicken thighs with salt and pepper, then brown on both sides, about 3 minutes per side.
3. Remove chicken from the pot and set aside.
4. Add quinoa, chicken broth, lemon juice, zest, garlic-infused oil, zucchini, bell pepper, and thyme to the pot. Stir to combine.
5. Return the chicken to the pot, placing it on top of the quinoa mixture.
6. Cover and simmer for 20 minutes or until the quinoa is cooked and the chicken is tender.

TIPS:

- Garnish with fresh parsley for added color and flavor.
- Serve with a side of steamed spinach for a complete meal.

N.V.: Calories: 350, Fat: 14g, Carbs: 34g, Protein: 25g, Sugar: 3g, Sodium: 320 mg, Potassium: 550 mg, Cholesterol: 90 mg

ONE-POT BEEF AND CABBAGE STIR-FRY

PREPARATION TIME: 10 min
COOKING TIME: 15 min
MODE OF COOKING: Stovetop
SERVINGS: 4
INGREDIENTS:

- 1 lb. ground beef (lean)
- 1/2 head of green cabbage, shredded
- 1 carrot, julienned
- 1 red bell pepper, sliced
- 1 Tbsp olive oil
- 2 Tbsp tamari (gluten-free soy sauce)
- 1 tsp garlic-infused olive oil
- Salt and pepper to taste
- Sesame seeds for garnish (optional)

DIRECTIONS:

1. Heat olive oil in a large skillet over medium heat.
2. Add ground beef, breaking it up as it cooks, and season with salt, pepper, and garlic-infused olive oil.
3. Once beef is browned, add cabbage, carrot, and bell pepper to the skillet. Stir-fry for 5 minutes until vegetables are tender-crisp.
4. Stir in tamari and cook for an additional 2 minutes.
5. Garnish with sesame seeds before serving, if desired.

TIPS:

- Serve with a side of rice or quinoa for a complete meal.
- Add a dash of rice vinegar for extra tanginess.

N.V.: Calories: 350, Fat: 20g, Carbs: 18g, Protein: 25g, Sugar: 6g, Sodium: 620 mg, Potassium: 700 mg, Cholesterol: 80 mg

ONE-POT CHICKEN AND VEGETABLE CURRY

PREPARATION TIME: 10 min
COOKING TIME: 20 min
MODE OF COOKING: Stovetop
SERVINGS: 4
INGREDIENTS:

- 4 boneless, skinless chicken thighs, cut into bite-sized pieces
- 1 cup coconut milk (canned, low-FODMAP)
- 1 cup low-sodium chicken broth
- 1 zucchini, diced
- 1 red bell pepper, diced
- 1 Tbsp olive oil
- 1 tsp curry powder
- 1/2 tsp turmeric
- 1 tsp garlic-infused olive oil
- Salt and pepper to taste
- Fresh cilantro for garnish

DIRECTIONS:

1. Heat olive oil in a large pot over medium heat.
2. Add chicken, seasoning with salt and pepper, and cook until browned, about 5 minutes.
3. Stir in zucchini, bell pepper, curry powder, turmeric, and garlic-infused oil.
4. Add coconut milk and chicken broth, stirring to combine.
5. Bring to a simmer, cover, and cook for 15 minutes, or until chicken is cooked through and vegetables are tender.
6. Garnish with fresh cilantro before serving.

TIPS:

- Serve with a side of steamed jasmine rice.
- For extra heat, add a pinch of cayenne pepper.

N.V.: Calories: 380, Fat: 24g, Carbs: 12g, Protein: 28g, Sugar: 3g, Sodium: 320 mg, Potassium: 600 mg, Cholesterol: 85 mg

ONE-POT GROUND BEEF AND POTATO HASH

PREPARATION TIME: 10 min
COOKING TIME: 20 min
MODE OF COOKING: Stovetop
SERVINGS: 4
INGREDIENTS:

- 1 lb. ground beef (lean)
- 4 small potatoes, diced
- 1 red bell pepper, diced
- 1 zucchini, diced
- 1 Tbsp olive oil
- 1 tsp paprika
- 1/2 tsp dried thyme
- Salt and pepper to taste
- Fresh parsley for garnish

DIRECTIONS:

1. Heat olive oil in a large skillet over medium heat.
2. Add ground beef, breaking it up as it cooks, and season with salt, pepper, paprika, and thyme.
3. Once beef is browned, add potatoes, bell pepper, and zucchini. Stir well.
4. Cover and cook for 15 minutes, stirring occasionally, until potatoes are tender.
5. Garnish with fresh parsley before serving.

TIPS:

- Serve with a side of eggs for a hearty breakfast or dinner.
- Add a sprinkle of grated cheddar cheese (lactose-free) for extra flavor.

N.V.: Calories: 420, Fat: 22g, Carbs: 30g, Protein: 28g, Sugar: 4g, Sodium: 350 mg, Potassium: 800 mg, Cholesterol: 90 mg

LOW-FODMAP MACARONI AND CHEESE

PREPARATION TIME: 10 min
COOKING TIME: 20 min
MODE OF COOKING: Stovetop/Baking
SERVINGS: 4

INGREDIENTS:

- 8 oz gluten-free elbow macaroni
- 2 cups lactose-free cheddar cheese, shredded
- 1 cup lactose-free milk
- 2 Tbsp gluten-free flour
- 2 Tbsp olive oil
- 1/2 tsp mustard powder
- Salt and pepper to taste
- 1/4 cup gluten-free breadcrumbs

DIRECTIONS:

1. Preheat oven to 350°F (175°C).
2. Cook gluten-free macaroni according to package instructions and set aside.
3. In a saucepan, heat olive oil over medium heat. Add gluten-free flour and mustard powder, stirring constantly for 1 minute.
4. Gradually whisk in lactose-free milk, continuing to stir until the mixture thickens.
5. Remove from heat and stir in shredded cheddar cheese until melted and smooth.
6. Combine the cheese sauce with the cooked macaroni and pour into a baking dish.
7. Top with gluten-free breadcrumbs and bake for 15 minutes, or until the top is golden.

TIPS:

- Add a sprinkle of smoked paprika or chives on top for added flavor.
- Serve with a side of roasted vegetables for a balanced meal.

N.V.: Calories: 480, Fat: 24g, Carbs: 48g, Protein: 18g, Sugar: 3g, Sodium: 520 mg, Potassium: 350 mg, Cholesterol: 60 mg

LOW-FODMAP CHICKEN ALFREDO

PREPARATION TIME: 10 min
COOKING TIME: 20 min
MODE OF COOKING: Stovetop
SERVINGS: 4
INGREDIENTS:

- 2 boneless, skinless chicken breasts, sliced into strips
- 8 oz gluten-free fettuccine
- 1 cup lactose-free heavy cream
- 1/2 cup lactose-free Parmesan cheese, grated
- 2 Tbsp olive oil
- 1 tsp garlic-infused olive oil
- 1/2 tsp dried thyme
- Salt and pepper to taste
- Fresh parsley for garnish

DIRECTIONS:

1. Cook gluten-free fettuccine according to package instructions. Drain and set aside.
2. Heat olive oil and garlic-infused olive oil in a large skillet over medium heat.
3. Add chicken strips, seasoning with salt, pepper, and thyme. Cook until golden brown and cooked through, about 5-7 minutes.
4. Reduce heat to low and stir in the lactose-free heavy cream and grated Parmesan. Simmer for 2-3 minutes until the sauce thickens.
5. Toss the cooked pasta with the sauce until well-coated.
6. Garnish with fresh parsley before serving.

TIPS:

- Add steamed spinach or zucchini for extra nutrients.
- Serve with a side of gluten-free garlic bread.

N.V.: Calories: 480, Fat: 26g, Carbs: 38g, Protein: 28g, Sugar: 2g, Sodium: 400 mg, Potassium: 300 mg, Cholesterol: 110 mg

LOW-FODMAP TURKEY MEATBALLS WITH MARINARA SAUCE

PREPARATION TIME: 10 min
COOKING TIME: 20 min
MODE OF COOKING: Stovetop/Baking
SERVINGS: 4
INGREDIENTS:

- 1 lb. ground turkey
- 1/2 cup gluten-free breadcrumbs
- 1 egg
- 1 tsp dried oregano
- 1/2 tsp dried basil
- Salt and pepper to taste
- 1 Tbsp olive oil
- 2 cups low-FODMAP marinara sauce
- 1/4 cup lactose-free Parmesan cheese, grated

DIRECTIONS:

1. Preheat oven to 375°F (190°C).
2. In a large bowl, mix ground turkey, gluten-free breadcrumbs, egg, oregano, basil, salt, and pepper. Form into small meatballs.
3. Heat olive oil in a large skillet over medium heat. Brown the meatballs on all sides for about 5 minutes.
4. Transfer meatballs to a baking dish, pour marinara sauce over them, and sprinkle with Parmesan cheese.
5. Bake for 15 minutes, or until meatballs are cooked through.

TIPS:

- Serve with gluten-free pasta or a side of steamed vegetables.
- Add fresh basil leaves for extra flavor.

N.V.: Calories: 320, Fat: 18g, Carbs: 16g, Protein: 28g, Sugar: 4g, Sodium: 480 mg, Potassium: 600 mg, Cholesterol: 100 mg

Low-FODMAP Beef Stroganoff

PREPARATION TIME: 10 min
COOKING TIME: 20 min
MODE OF COOKING: Stovetop
SERVINGS: 4
INGREDIENTS:

- 1 lb. beef sirloin, thinly sliced
- 8 oz gluten-free pasta
- 1 cup lactose-free sour cream
- 1/2 cup low-sodium beef broth
- 1 Tbsp gluten-free flour
- 2 Tbsp olive oil
- 1 tsp garlic-infused olive oil
- 1 tsp dried thyme
- Salt and pepper to taste

DIRECTIONS:

1. Cook gluten-free pasta according to package instructions. Drain and set aside.
2. In a large skillet, heat olive oil over medium heat. Add beef slices and cook until browned, about 5 minutes. Remove from skillet and set aside.
3. In the same skillet, add gluten-free flour, cooking for 1 minute. Gradually add beef broth, stirring until thickened.
4. Stir in lactose-free sour cream, garlic-infused olive oil, thyme, salt, and pepper.
5. Return beef to the skillet and cook for an additional 5 minutes, until heated through.
6. Toss the beef and sauce with the cooked pasta.

TIPS:

- Garnish with fresh parsley for added flavor.
- Serve with a side of steamed green beans or roasted carrots.

N.V.: Calories: 450, Fat: 24g, Carbs: 32g, Protein: 28g, Sugar: 3g, Sodium: 400 mg, Potassium: 700 mg, Cholesterol: 90 mg

Low-FODMAP Chicken and Spinach Frittata

PREPARATION TIME: 10 min
COOKING TIME: 20 min
MODE OF COOKING: Baking
SERVINGS: 4
INGREDIENTS:

- 6 large eggs
- 2 boneless, skinless chicken breasts, cooked and diced
- 2 cups fresh spinach
- 1/2 cup lactose-free cheddar cheese, shredded
- 1/4 cup lactose-free milk
- 1 tsp garlic-infused olive oil
- 1 Tbsp olive oil
- Salt and pepper to taste

DIRECTIONS:

1. Preheat oven to 375°F (190°C).
2. In a large bowl, whisk together eggs, lactose-free milk, garlic-infused olive oil, salt, and pepper.
3. Heat olive oil in an oven-safe skillet over medium heat. Add spinach and cook until wilted, about 2 minutes.
4. Add cooked chicken to the skillet and pour the egg mixture over it.
5. Sprinkle with shredded cheddar cheese.
6. Transfer the skillet to the oven and bake for 15 minutes, or until the frittata is set and golden brown on top.

TIPS:

- Serve with a side salad or gluten-free toast.
- Add fresh herbs like parsley or chives for extra flavor.

N.V.: Calories: 320, Fat: 20g, Carbs: 4g, Protein: 30g, Sugar: 1g, Sodium: 380 mg, Potassium: 450 mg, Cholesterol: 310 mg

Low-FODMAP Chicken and Vegetable Stir-Fry

PREPARATION TIME: 10 min
COOKING TIME: 15 min
MODE OF COOKING: Stir-Frying
SERVINGS: 4
INGREDIENTS:
- 2 boneless, skinless chicken breasts, sliced into thin strips
- 1 red bell pepper, sliced
- 1 zucchini, sliced
- 1 cup carrots, julienned
- 2 Tbsp tamari (gluten-free soy sauce)
- 1 Tbsp sesame oil
- 1 tsp garlic-infused olive oil
- 1 tsp grated ginger
- 1 Tbsp olive oil
- Salt and pepper to taste

DIRECTIONS:
1. Heat olive oil in a large skillet or wok over medium heat.
2. Add chicken strips and cook until browned, about 5 minutes.
3. Remove chicken from the skillet and set aside.
4. In the same skillet, add garlic-infused olive oil, grated ginger, bell pepper, zucchini, and carrots. Stir-fry for 5 minutes until vegetables are tender-crisp.
5. Return chicken to the skillet, add tamari and sesame oil, and stir to combine. Cook for an additional 2 minutes until everything is well-coated and heated through.

TIPS:
- Serve over rice or quinoa for a complete meal.
- Garnish with sesame seeds or chopped green onions for extra flavor.

N.V.: Calories: 300, Fat: 14g, Carbs: 18g, Protein: 25g, Sugar: 4g, Sodium: 500 mg, Potassium: 600 mg, Cholesterol: 70 mg

CHAPTER 8: VEGETARIAN AND VEGAN CHOICES

Embarking on a low-FODMAP journey doesn't mean you have to compromise on the richness and diversity of vegetarian or vegan cuisine. In fact, adapting to a diet sensitive to such needs can open up a delightful world of culinary exploration that respects both your health and your taste buds. This chapter is dedicated to those who cherish plant-based diets, offering enticing dishes where flavor and variety shine, all within the gentle boundaries set by low-FODMAP guidelines.

As we delve into the vegetarian and vegan recipes, you'll discover how bountiful and satisfying plant-based meals can be even under the constraints of a low-FODMAP diet. The key lies in knowing your ingredients well and harnessing their potential to create dishes that are both nourishing and delicious. For example, tofu and tempeh will become your trusted proteins, versatile enough to be transformed into exotic-spiced curries or comforting scrambles that are friendly to your digestive system.

Navigating through a plant-based lifestyle on a low-FODMAP diet also means mastering the art of substitution and innovation. You'll learn to swap high-FODMAP offenders like garlic and onions with asafetida or chives, infusing meals with the depth of flavor that every satisfying dish deserves. This isn't just about removing ingredients that trigger symptoms; it's about reimagining your plate and discovering new favorites in a way that still adheres to dietary needs.

And it's more than just recipes. This chapter serves as a beacon for those seeking inspiration in the often-murky waters of dietary restrictions. It's about embracing your creative instincts in the kitchen, experimenting with hearty vegetable-based mains and snacks, and perhaps most importantly, enjoying the process. Our plant-based journey in this low-FODMAP landscape ensures you're well-equipped with the practical knowledge needed to eat well every day without feeling restricted.

Join me, as we prove that with a bit of know-how and a lot of passion, maintaining a vegetarian or vegan lifestyle on a low-FODMAP diet isn't just manageable; it's an exciting, flavor-filled adventure.

TEMPEH STIR-FRY WITH VEGETABLES

PREPARATION TIME: 10 min
COOKING TIME: 15 min
MODE OF COOKING: Stir-Frying
SERVINGS: 4
INGREDIENTS:

- 1 block tempeh, sliced into thin strips
- 1 red bell pepper, sliced
- 1 zucchini, sliced
- 1 carrot, julienned
- 2 Tbsp tamari (gluten-free soy sauce)
- 1 Tbsp olive oil
- 1 tsp garlic-infused olive oil
- 1 tsp grated ginger
- 1 tsp sesame oil (optional)

DIRECTIONS:

1. Heat olive oil in a large skillet over medium heat.
2. Add tempeh slices and cook until golden on both sides, about 5 minutes.
3. Remove tempeh from the skillet and set aside.
4. In the same skillet, add garlic-infused olive oil, ginger, bell pepper, zucchini, and carrot. Stir-fry for 5 minutes until vegetables are tender-crisp.
5. Return tempeh to the skillet and add tamari. Stir to combine and cook for an additional 2 minutes.
6. Drizzle with sesame oil before serving, if desired.

TIPS:

- Serve over rice or quinoa for a complete meal.
- Garnish with chopped green onions or sesame seeds for added flavor.

N.V.: Calories: 300, Fat: 18g, Carbs: 20g, Protein: 20g, Sugar: 4g, Sodium: 450 mg, Potassium: 400 mg, Cholesterol: 0 mg

CRISPY BAKED TOFU WITH LEMON AND HERBS

PREPARATION TIME: 10 min
COOKING TIME: 20 min
MODE OF COOKING: Baking
SERVINGS: 4
INGREDIENTS:

- 1 block firm tofu, pressed and cubed
- 2 Tbsp olive oil
- 1 lemon, juiced and zested
- 1 tsp dried oregano
- 1 tsp dried thyme
- Salt and pepper to taste
- 1 tsp garlic-infused olive oil (optional)

DIRECTIONS:

1. Preheat oven to 400°F (204°C).
2. In a bowl, toss the cubed tofu with olive oil, lemon juice, zest, oregano, thyme, salt, and pepper.
3. Spread the tofu cubes on a baking sheet lined with parchment paper.
4. Bake for 20 minutes, turning halfway through, until tofu is golden and crispy.

TIPS:

- Serve over a bed of quinoa or with steamed vegetables for a complete meal.
- Add a drizzle of additional lemon juice before serving for extra zing.

N.V.: Calories: 220, Fat: 14g, Carbs: 8g, Protein: 16g, Sugar: 1g, Sodium: 15 mg, Potassium: 210 mg, Cholesterol: 0 mg

TEMPEH TACOS WITH AVOCADO

PREPARATION TIME: 10 min
COOKING TIME: 10 min
MODE OF COOKING: Stovetop
SERVINGS: 4
INGREDIENTS:

- 1 block tempeh, crumbled
- 1 avocado, sliced
- 1 red bell pepper, diced
- 1 tsp cumin
- 1 tsp smoked paprika

- 2 Tbsp olive oil
- 1/2 cup lactose-free sour cream
- Salt and pepper to taste
- 8 small gluten-free tortillas

DIRECTIONS:

1. Heat olive oil in a large skillet over medium heat.
2. Add crumbled tempeh, cumin, smoked paprika, salt, and pepper. Cook for 5 minutes until tempeh is heated through and slightly crispy.
3. Warm the tortillas in a dry skillet or microwave.
4. Fill each tortilla with tempeh, diced bell pepper, and avocado slices.
5. Top with a dollop of lactose-free sour cream.

TIPS:

- Add a squeeze of lime juice over the tacos for a fresh burst of flavor.
- Serve with a side of gluten-free tortilla chips and salsa.

N.V.: Calories: 370, Fat: 22g, Carbs: 32g, Protein: 14g, Sugar: 3g, Sodium: 340 mg, Potassium: 600 mg, Cholesterol: 0 mg

TOFU SCRAMBLE WITH SPINACH AND TOMATOES

PREPARATION TIME: 5 min
COOKING TIME: 10 min
MODE OF COOKING: Stovetop
SERVINGS: 4
INGREDIENTS:

- 1 block firm tofu, crumbled
- 2 cups fresh spinach
- 1 cup cherry tomatoes, halved
- 1 Tbsp olive oil
- 1 tsp turmeric
- 1 tsp garlic-infused olive oil
- Salt and pepper to taste

DIRECTIONS:

1. Heat olive oil in a large skillet over medium heat.
2. Add crumbled tofu, turmeric, garlic-infused olive oil, salt, and pepper.

Cook for 5 minutes, stirring frequently.
3. Add spinach and cherry tomatoes to the skillet, cooking until spinach is wilted and tomatoes are softened, about 3 minutes.
4. Serve hot, garnished with fresh herbs if desired.

TIPS:

- Serve with gluten-free toast or a side of roasted potatoes.
- Add a sprinkle of nutritional yeast for a cheesy flavor.

N.V.: Calories: 200, Fat: 12g, Carbs: 8g, Protein: 16g, Sugar: 2g, Sodium: 150 mg, Potassium: 600 mg, Cholesterol: 0 mg

TEMPEH FAJITAS WITH PEPPERS AND ONIONS

PREPARATION TIME: 10 min
COOKING TIME: 15 min
MODE OF COOKING: Stovetop
SERVINGS: 4
INGREDIENTS:

- 1 block tempeh, sliced into strips
- 1 red bell pepper, sliced
- 1 yellow bell pepper, sliced
- 1 red onion, sliced (use only if low-FODMAP or substitute with more bell pepper)
- 1 Tbsp olive oil
- 1 tsp cumin
- 1 tsp smoked paprika
- 1/2 tsp chili powder
- Salt and pepper to taste
- 8 small gluten-free tortillas

DIRECTIONS:

1. Heat olive oil in a large skillet over medium heat.
2. Add tempeh strips and cook until golden, about 5 minutes.
3. Add bell peppers, onion (if using), cumin, smoked paprika, chili powder, salt, and pepper. Stir-fry for 8-10 minutes until vegetables are tender.

4. Warm the tortillas in a dry skillet or microwave.
5. Serve the tempeh and vegetable mixture in tortillas.

TIPS:
- Serve with lactose-free sour cream and guacamole.
- Add a squeeze of lime juice for extra freshness.

N.V.: Calories: 340, Fat: 18g, Carbs: 30g, Protein: 18g, Sugar: 4g, Sodium: 380 mg, Potassium: 500 mg, Cholesterol: 0 mg

MAPLE-SOY GLAZED TOFU

PREPARATION TIME: 10 min
COOKING TIME: 15 min
MODE OF COOKING: Stovetop
SERVINGS: 4
INGREDIENTS:
- 1 block firm tofu, pressed and cubed
- 2 Tbsp tamari (gluten-free soy sauce)
- 1 Tbsp maple syrup
- 1 Tbsp rice vinegar
- 1 Tbsp sesame oil
- 1 tsp garlic-infused olive oil
- 1 tsp grated ginger
- 1 Tbsp olive oil

DIRECTIONS:
1. Heat olive oil in a large skillet over medium heat.
2. Add tofu cubes and cook until golden on all sides, about 5 minutes.
3. In a small bowl, whisk together tamari, maple syrup, rice vinegar, sesame oil, garlic-infused olive oil, and ginger.
4. Pour the sauce over the tofu, stirring to coat evenly.
5. Cook for an additional 5 minutes, until the sauce is thickened and the tofu is well-glazed.

TIPS:
- Serve over rice or quinoa with steamed broccoli.
- Garnish with sesame seeds or chopped green onions for added flavor.

N.V.: Calories: 240, Fat: 14g, Carbs: 16g, Protein: 14g, Sugar: 5g, Sodium: 360 mg, Potassium: 250 mg, Cholesterol: 0 mg

ZUCCHINI NOODLES WITH PESTO AND CHERRY TOMATOES

PREPARATION TIME: 10 min
COOKING TIME: 10 min
MODE OF COOKING: Stovetop
SERVINGS: 4
INGREDIENTS:
- 4 medium zucchinis, spiralized into noodles
- 1 cup cherry tomatoes, halved
- 1/4 cup lactose-free Parmesan cheese, grated
- 1/4 cup pine nuts
- 1/4 cup fresh basil leaves
- 2 Tbsp olive oil
- 1 tsp garlic-infused olive oil
- Salt and pepper to taste

DIRECTIONS:
1. Heat olive oil and garlic-infused olive oil in a large skillet over medium heat.
2. Add zucchini noodles and sauté for 3-4 minutes until tender.
3. In a food processor, blend basil, pine nuts, Parmesan cheese, and a pinch of salt to make the pesto.
4. Toss zucchini noodles with the pesto and cherry tomatoes in the skillet until well combined.
5. Season with salt and pepper to taste.

TIPS:
- Serve with a side of gluten-free bread for a heartier meal.
- Garnish with extra Parmesan and fresh basil.

N.V.: Calories: 280, Fat: 20g, Carbs: 16g, Protein: 10g, Sugar: 6g, Sodium: 240 mg, Potassium: 550 mg, Cholesterol: 10 mg

ROASTED VEGETABLE AND QUINOA BOWL

PREPARATION TIME: 10 min
COOKING TIME: 20 min
MODE OF COOKING: Roasting/Stovetop
SERVINGS: 4
INGREDIENTS:

- 1 cup quinoa, rinsed
- 2 cups low-sodium vegetable broth
- 1 red bell pepper, diced
- 1 zucchini, diced
- 1 carrot, diced
- 1 sweet potato, diced
- 2 Tbsp olive oil
- 1 tsp dried thyme
- Salt and pepper to taste
- Fresh parsley for garnish

DIRECTIONS:

1. Preheat oven to 400°F (204°C).
2. Toss diced red bell pepper, zucchini, carrot, and sweet potato with olive oil, thyme, salt, and pepper.
3. Spread the vegetables on a baking sheet and roast for 20 minutes until tender and slightly caramelized.
4. Meanwhile, bring vegetable broth to a boil in a medium pot. Add quinoa, reduce heat, and simmer for 15 minutes until the quinoa is cooked and the liquid is absorbed.
5. Combine the roasted vegetables with the cooked quinoa in a large bowl. Mix well.
6. Garnish with fresh parsley before serving.

TIPS:

- Add a squeeze of lemon juice for a burst of freshness.
- Serve with a side of avocado slices for added creaminess.

N.V.: Calories: 380, Fat: 14g, Carbs: 55g, Protein: 10g, Sugar: 10g, Sodium: 300 mg, Potassium: 900 mg, Cholesterol: 0 mg

GRILLED VEGETABLE SKEWERS WITH QUINOA

PREPARATION TIME: 10 min
COOKING TIME: 20 min
MODE OF COOKING: Grilling
SERVINGS: 4
INGREDIENTS:

- 1 red bell pepper, cut into chunks
- 1 zucchini, sliced
- 1 yellow squash, sliced
- 1 red onion, cut into chunks (optional, if tolerated)
- 1-pint cherry tomatoes
- 1 cup quinoa, rinsed
- 2 cups low-sodium vegetable broth
- 2 Tbsp olive oil
- 1 tsp dried oregano
- Salt and pepper to taste

DIRECTIONS:

1. Preheat grill to medium heat.
2. In a bowl, toss bell pepper, zucchini, yellow squash, red onion, and cherry tomatoes with olive oil, oregano, salt, and pepper.
3. Thread the vegetables onto skewers.
4. Grill the skewers for 8-10 minutes, turning occasionally, until vegetables are tender and slightly charred.
5. While the vegetables are grilling, cook quinoa in vegetable broth according to package instructions.
6. Serve the grilled vegetable skewers over a bed of quinoa.

TIPS:

- Serve with a side of hummus or a simple vinaigrette.
- Garnish with fresh herbs like parsley or cilantro.

N.V.: Calories: 320, Fat: 12g, Carbs: 45g, Protein: 8g, Sugar: 7g, Sodium: 300 mg, Potassium: 700 mg, Cholesterol: 0 mg

ROASTED VEGETABLE AND LENTIL SALAD

PREPARATION TIME: 10 min
COOKING TIME: 20 min
MODE OF COOKING: Roasting
SERVINGS: 4
INGREDIENTS:

- 1 cup cooked lentils (ensure they are low-FODMAP)
- 1 red bell pepper, diced
- 1 zucchini, diced
- 1 carrot, diced
- 1 sweet potato, diced
- 2 Tbsp olive oil
- 1 tsp dried oregano
- 1 tsp smoked paprika
- Salt and pepper to taste
- 2 cups fresh spinach, chopped
- 1/4 cup lactose-free feta cheese, crumbled

DIRECTIONS:

1. Preheat oven to 400°F (204°C).
2. Toss diced red bell pepper, zucchini, carrot, and sweet potato with olive oil, oregano, smoked paprika, salt, and pepper.
3. Spread the vegetables on a baking sheet and roast for 20 minutes until tender and slightly caramelized.
4. In a large bowl, combine roasted vegetables, cooked lentils, and chopped spinach.
5. Top with crumbled feta cheese before serving.

TIPS:

- Serve with a side of gluten-free bread.
- Add a drizzle of balsamic glaze for extra flavor.

N.V.: Calories: 360, Fat: 14g, Carbs: 50g, Protein: 12g, Sugar: 10g, Sodium: 400 mg, Potassium: 850 mg, Cholesterol: 20 mg

GRILLED EGGPLANT AND ZUCCHINI STACK WITH TOMATO AND BASIL

PREPARATION TIME: 10 min
COOKING TIME: 15 min
MODE OF COOKING: Grilling
SERVINGS: 4
INGREDIENTS:

- 2 medium eggplants, sliced into rounds
- 2 zucchinis, sliced into rounds
- 2 large tomatoes, sliced
- 1/4 cup lactose-free mozzarella cheese, shredded
- 1/4 cup fresh basil leaves
- 2 Tbsp olive oil
- 1 tsp balsamic vinegar
- Salt and pepper to taste

DIRECTIONS:

1. Preheat grill to medium-high heat.
2. Brush eggplant and zucchini slices with olive oil, and season with salt and pepper.
3. Grill the eggplant and zucchini slices for about 3-4 minutes on each side, until tender and slightly charred.
4. Layer the grilled eggplant and zucchini slices with tomato slices, mozzarella cheese, and fresh basil leaves, stacking them to create a tower.
5. Drizzle with balsamic vinegar before serving.

TIPS:

- Serve with a side of gluten-free garlic bread.
- Garnish with additional fresh basil or a sprinkle of lactose-free Parmesan cheese.

N.V.: Calories: 240, Fat: 16g, Carbs: 18g, Protein: 6g, Sugar: 9g, Sodium: 150 mg, Potassium: 700 mg, Cholesterol: 10 mg

SWEET POTATO AND BLACK BEAN TACOS

PREPARATION TIME: 10 min
COOKING TIME: 20 min
MODE OF COOKING: Stovetop
SERVINGS: 4
INGREDIENTS:

- 2 large sweet potatoes, peeled and diced
- 1 can black beans, drained and rinsed (ensure they are low-FODMAP)
- 8 small gluten-free tortillas
- 1 tsp cumin
- 1 tsp smoked paprika
- 1/2 tsp chili powder
- 2 Tbsp olive oil
- 1/4 cup lactose-free sour cream
- 1 avocado, sliced
- Fresh cilantro for garnish
- Salt and pepper to taste

DIRECTIONS:

1. In a large skillet, heat olive oil over medium heat. Add diced sweet potatoes and cook for 10 minutes until they begin to soften.
2. Add cumin, smoked paprika, chili powder, salt, and pepper. Stir to coat the sweet potatoes evenly with the spices.
3. Add black beans to the skillet and cook for an additional 5 minutes until heated through.
4. Warm the gluten-free tortillas in a dry skillet or microwave.
5. Fill each tortilla with the sweet potato and black bean mixture. Top with avocado slices, a dollop of lactose-free sour cream, and fresh cilantro.

TIPS:

- Serve with a side of lime wedges for a fresh squeeze of citrus.
- Add a sprinkle of lactose-free cheese if desired.

N.V.: Calories: 380, Fat: 14g, Carbs: 58g, Protein: 10g, Sugar: 8g, Sodium: 400 mg, Potassium: 900 mg, Cholesterol: 0 mg

SPICY ROASTED CHICKPEAS

PREPARATION TIME: 5 min
COOKING TIME: 25 min
MODE OF COOKING: Roasting
SERVINGS: 4
INGREDIENTS:

- 1 can chickpeas, drained and rinsed (ensure they are low-FODMAP)
- 2 Tbsp olive oil
- 1 tsp smoked paprika
- 1/2 tsp cumin
- 1/2 tsp chili powder
- Salt and pepper to taste

DIRECTIONS:

1. Preheat oven to 400°F (204°C).
2. Pat chickpeas dry with a paper towel to remove excess moisture.
3. In a bowl, toss chickpeas with olive oil, smoked paprika, cumin, chili powder, salt, and pepper.
4. Spread the chickpeas in a single layer on a baking sheet.
5. Roast for 20-25 minutes, shaking the pan halfway through, until chickpeas are crispy and golden brown.

TIPS:

- Store in an airtight container for up to a week for a quick snack.
- Add to salads for extra crunch.

N.V.: Calories: 180, Fat: 8g, Carbs: 22g, Protein: 6g, Sugar: 1g, Sodium: 180 mg, Potassium: 200 mg, Cholesterol: 0 mg

BAKED SWEET POTATO FRIES

PREPARATION TIME: 10 min
COOKING TIME: 20 min
MODE OF COOKING: Baking
SERVINGS: 4
INGREDIENTS:

- 2 large sweet potatoes, peeled and cut into thin fries
- 2 Tbsp olive oil
- 1 tsp smoked paprika
- 1/2 tsp garlic-infused olive oil
- Salt and pepper to taste

DIRECTIONS:

1. Preheat oven to 425°F (218°C).
2. In a bowl, toss sweet potato fries with olive oil, smoked paprika, garlic-infused olive oil, salt, and pepper.
3. Spread fries in a single layer on a baking sheet lined with parchment paper.
4. Bake for 20 minutes, flipping halfway through, until fries are crispy and golden.

TIPS:

- Serve with a vegan dipping sauce like tahini or avocado dip.
- Sprinkle with fresh herbs like parsley or cilantro for added flavor.

N.V.: Calories: 200, Fat: 10g, Carbs: 28g, Protein: 2g, Sugar: 6g, Sodium: 150 mg, Potassium: 400 mg, Cholesterol: 0 mg

VEGAN GUACAMOLE AND VEGGIE STICKS

PREPARATION TIME: 10 min
COOKING TIME: None
MODE OF COOKING: No Cooking
SERVINGS: 4
INGREDIENTS:

- 2 ripe avocados
- 1 lime, juiced
- 1/4 cup fresh cilantro, chopped
- 1 tsp garlic-infused olive oil
- Salt and pepper to taste
- 1 cucumber, cut into sticks
- 2 carrots, cut into sticks
- 1 red bell pepper, cut into sticks

DIRECTIONS:

1. In a bowl, mash the avocados with a fork.
2. Stir in lime juice, cilantro, garlic-infused olive oil, salt, and pepper.
3. Serve the guacamole with cucumber, carrot, and red bell pepper sticks.

TIPS:

- Add a pinch of smoked paprika or chili flakes to the guacamole for extra spice.
- Serve as a snack or appetizer at gatherings.

N.V.: Calories: 150, Fat: 12g, Carbs: 10g, Protein: 2g, Sugar: 2g, Sodium: 120 mg, Potassium: 450 mg, Cholesterol: 0 mg

CRISPY KALE CHIPS

PREPARATION TIME: 5 min
COOKING TIME: 15 min
MODE OF COOKING: Baking
SERVINGS: 4
INGREDIENTS:

- 1 bunch of kale, stems removed and torn into bite-sized pieces
- 2 Tbsp olive oil
- 1 tsp smoked paprika
- Salt and pepper to taste

DIRECTIONS:

1. Preheat oven to 350°F (175°C).
2. In a bowl, toss kale pieces with olive oil, smoked paprika, salt, and pepper.
3. Spread the kale in a single layer on a baking sheet lined with parchment paper.
4. Bake for 12-15 minutes, until the kale is crispy but not burnt.

TIPS:

- Watch the kale carefully towards the end of the cooking time to prevent burning.
- Experiment with different seasonings like nutritional yeast for a cheesy flavor.

N.V.: Calories: 90, Fat: 7g, Carbs: 7g, Protein: 2g, Sugar: 0g, Sodium: 100 mg, Potassium: 300 mg, Cholesterol: 0 mg

VEGAN ZUCCHINI FRITTERS

PREPARATION TIME: 10 min
COOKING TIME: 15 min
MODE OF COOKING: Pan-Frying
SERVINGS: 4
INGREDIENTS:

- 2 medium zucchinis, grated
- 1/4 cup gluten-free flour
- 2 Tbsp ground flaxseed mixed with 6 Tbsp water (as an egg replacer)
- 1/4 cup green onions, finely chopped (use only if tolerated)
- 1 tsp garlic-infused olive oil
- Salt and pepper to taste
- Olive oil for frying

DIRECTIONS:

1. In a bowl, mix grated zucchini with a pinch of salt. Let sit for 5 minutes, then squeeze out the excess moisture.
2. In another bowl, combine the grated zucchini, gluten-free flour, flaxseed mixture, green onions (if using), garlic-infused olive oil, salt, and pepper.
3. Heat olive oil in a skillet over medium heat.
4. Drop spoonfuls of the zucchini mixture into the skillet and flatten slightly with a spatula.
5. Cook for 3-4 minutes on each side until golden brown and crispy.
6. Drain on paper towels before serving.

TIPS:

- Serve with a vegan dipping sauce like tahini or avocado dip.

- Add a squeeze of lemon juice for a fresh flavor boost.

N.V.: Calories: 140, Fat: 8g, Carbs: 14g, Protein: 3g, Sugar: 3g, Sodium: 150 mg, Potassium: 400 mg, Cholesterol: 0 mg

VEGAN AVOCADO TOAST WITH RADISHES AND SESAME SEEDS

PREPARATION TIME: 5 min
COOKING TIME: None
MODE OF COOKING: No Cooking
SERVINGS: 2
INGREDIENTS:

- 1 ripe avocado
- 2 slices of gluten-free bread, toasted
- 4 radishes, thinly sliced
- 1 tsp sesame seeds
- 1 Tbsp lemon juice
- Salt and pepper to taste
- Fresh cilantro for garnish

DIRECTIONS:

1. In a small bowl, mash the avocado with lemon juice, salt, and pepper until smooth.
2. Spread the avocado mixture evenly on the toasted gluten-free bread slices.
3. Top with thinly sliced radishes and a sprinkle of sesame seeds.
4. Garnish with fresh cilantro before serving.

TIPS:

- Add a pinch of red pepper flakes for a spicy kick.
- Serve with a side of fresh fruit for a complete breakfast or snack.

N.V.: Calories: 220, Fat: 14g, Carbs: 20g, Protein: 4g, Sugar: 1g, Sodium: 180 mg, Potassium: 500 mg, Cholesterol: 0 mg

CHAPTER 9: SNACKS AND APPETIZERS

Welcome to the delightful world of snacks and appetizers, where each bite is not just a treat to your taste buds but also a caring embrace to your digestive system. Imagine hosting a party or simply enjoying a quiet evening at home, with dishes that are as kind to your gut as they are enticing to the eye. This chapter is dedicated to transforming the often-daunting world of the low-FODMAP diet into a playground of flavorsome, simple-to-make starters that ensure you never feel left out of culinary festivities.

The quest for gut-friendly appetizers can sometimes seem like navigating a maze confusing and a little intimidating. It's all too easy to rely on the same handful of recipes, leading to the very monotony you hoped to escape when you set out on your low-FODMAP journey. Through my own experiences and those shared by others with sensitive digestive systems, I've gathered insights and inspirations that promise to keep your snack trays vibrant and varied.

We'll embark on a culinary adventure that spans quick solo snacks like herbed cheese-stuffed peppers to crowd-pleasers such as a savory low-FODMAP salsa that no one will guess is diet-specific. These recipes are crafted to ensure that you can whip them up in moments of unexpected hunger or plan them for elaborate gatherings without fretting over your symptoms.

Remember, the fundamental goal of these recipes is not just to alleviate the potential physical discomfort but to also dissolve the psychological barriers associated with a therapeutic diet. The confidence to throw together a couple of ingredients and come up with something delectable and safe is empowering. It's about reclaiming the joy of casual dining and social engagements without the shadow of worry.

Through creative uses of low-FODMAP vegetables, grains, and proteins, and by harnessing the natural flavors of herbs and spices, these appetizers are designed to delight. They are more than just food; they are conversation starters, they are pieces of reassurance that delicious, pain-free eating is wonderfully possible. Let's turn what could be a restriction into a celebration of all the amazing foods you can enjoy.

QUICK VEGGIE WRAP

PREPARATION TIME: 10 min
COOKING TIME: None
MODE OF COOKING: No Cooking
SERVINGS: 2
INGREDIENTS:

- 2 gluten-free tortillas
- 1/2 cup hummus (ensure it's low-FODMAP)
- 1/2 cucumber, sliced into strips
- 1 carrot, grated
- 1/2 avocado, sliced
- 1/4 cup fresh spinach leaves
- Salt and pepper to taste

DIRECTIONS:

1. Spread hummus evenly over each tortilla.
2. Layer with cucumber, carrot, avocado, and spinach.
3. Season with salt and pepper, then roll up the tortillas tightly.
4. Slice in half and serve immediately.

TIPS:

- Add a squeeze of lemon juice for extra freshness.
- Serve with a side of fruit or a small salad for a more filling snack.

N.V.: Calories: 220, Fat: 12g, Carbs: 24g, Protein: 6g, Sugar: 4g, Sodium: 200 mg, Potassium: 400 mg, Cholesterol: 0 mg

GREEK YOGURT WITH BERRIES AND ALMONDS

PREPARATION TIME: 5 min
COOKING TIME: None
MODE OF COOKING: No Cooking
SERVINGS: 2
INGREDIENTS:

- 1 cup lactose-free Greek yogurt
- 1/2 cup fresh blueberries
- 1/2 cup fresh strawberries, sliced
- 2 Tbsp sliced almonds
- 1 tsp maple syrup (optional)

DIRECTIONS:

1. Divide the Greek yogurt between two serving bowls.
2. Top each bowl with blueberries, strawberries, and sliced almonds.
3. Drizzle with maple syrup if desired.

TIPS:

- Substitute with other low-FODMAP fruits like grapes or bananas if preferred.
- Add a sprinkle of chia seeds for extra fiber.

N.V.: Calories: 220, Fat: 10g, Carbs: 22g, Protein: 12g, Sugar: 12g, Sodium: 60 mg, Potassium: 350 mg, Cholesterol: 10 mg

QUICK AVOCADO TOAST WITH TOMATO

PREPARATION TIME: 5 min
COOKING TIME: None
MODE OF COOKING: No Cooking
SERVINGS: 2
INGREDIENTS:

- 1 ripe avocado
- 2 slices gluten-free bread, toasted
- 1 small tomato, sliced
- 1 Tbsp lemon juice
- Salt and pepper to taste
- Fresh basil for garnish

DIRECTIONS:

1. In a small bowl, mash the avocado with lemon juice, salt, and pepper.
2. Spread the avocado mixture evenly on the toasted gluten-free bread slices.
3. Top with tomato slices and garnish with fresh basil.

TIPS:

- Add a sprinkle of red pepper flakes for a spicy kick.
- Serve with a side of fresh fruit for a balanced snack.

N.V.: Calories: 240, Fat: 14g, Carbs: 24g, Protein: 4g, Sugar: 2g, Sodium: 180 mg, Potassium: 500 mg, Cholesterol: 0 mg

CUCUMBER AND HUMMUS BITES

PREPARATION TIME: 5 min
COOKING TIME: None
MODE OF COOKING: No Cooking
SERVINGS: 4
INGREDIENTS:
- 1 large cucumber, sliced into rounds
- 1/2 cup low-FODMAP hummus
- 1 Tbsp fresh dill, chopped
- 1 tsp lemon zest
- Salt and pepper to taste

DIRECTIONS:
1. Arrange the cucumber slices on a serving platter.
2. Top each slice with a small dollop of hummus.
3. Sprinkle with fresh dill, lemon zest, salt, and pepper.

TIPS:
- Add a sprinkle of paprika for extra flavor.
- Serve as a refreshing snack or light appetizer.

N.V.: Calories: 60, Fat: 3g, Carbs: 7g, Protein: 2g, Sugar: 2g, Sodium: 120 mg, Potassium: 150 mg, Cholesterol: 0 mg

QUICK GUACAMOLE WITH TORTILLA CHIPS

PREPARATION TIME: 5 min
COOKING TIME: None
MODE OF COOKING: No Cooking
SERVINGS: 2
INGREDIENTS:
- 2 ripe avocados
- 1 lime, juiced
- 1 Tbsp fresh cilantro, chopped
- 1/2 tsp garlic-infused olive oil
- Salt and pepper to taste
- 1 cup gluten-free tortilla chips

DIRECTIONS:
1. In a bowl, mash the avocados with a fork.
2. Stir in lime juice, cilantro, garlic-infused olive oil, salt, and pepper.
3. Serve the guacamole with gluten-free tortilla chips.

TIPS:
- Add a pinch of cumin or chili powder for extra flavor.
- Serve with a side of fresh salsa for a more complete snack.

N.V.: Calories: 220, Fat: 18g, Carbs: 18g, Protein: 3g, Sugar: 1g, Sodium: 140 mg, Potassium: 500 mg, Cholesterol: 0 mg

ZUCCHINI CHIPS

PREPARATION TIME: 5 min
COOKING TIME: 15 min
MODE OF COOKING: Baking
SERVINGS: 4
INGREDIENTS:
- 1 large zucchini, thinly sliced
- 1 Tbsp olive oil
- 1/4 tsp salt
- 1/4 tsp black pepper
- 1/4 tsp smoked paprika (optional)

DIRECTIONS:
1. Preheat oven to 400°F (200°C). Line a baking sheet with parchment paper.
2. In a bowl, toss the zucchini slices with olive oil, salt, pepper, and smoked paprika if using.
3. Arrange the slices in a single layer on the prepared baking sheet.
4. Bake for 15 minutes or until crisp and golden, turning once halfway through.
5. Allow to cool slightly before serving.

TIPS:
- Serve with a side of lactose-free Greek yogurt dip for added flavor.
- These chips are best enjoyed fresh but can be stored in an airtight container for up to 2 days.

N.V.: Calories: 50, Fat: 4g, Carbs: 4g, Protein: 1g, Sugar: 2g, Sodium: 120 mg, Potassium: 200 mg, Cholesterol: 0 mg

STUFFED MINI BELL PEPPERS WITH HERBED GOAT CHEESE

PREPARATION TIME: 10 min
COOKING TIME: None
MODE OF COOKING: No Cooking
SERVINGS: 4
INGREDIENTS:

- 12 mini bell peppers, halved and seeded
- 4 oz lactose-free goat cheese
- 2 Tbsp fresh chives, chopped
- 2 Tbsp fresh parsley, chopped
- 1 tsp lemon zest
- 1 Tbsp olive oil
- Salt and pepper to taste

DIRECTIONS:

1. In a small bowl, mix the lactose-free goat cheese with chives, parsley, lemon zest, olive oil, salt, and pepper until well combined.
2. Fill each mini bell pepper half with the goat cheese mixture.
3. Arrange on a platter and serve immediately.

TIPS:

- For added flavor, drizzle with a bit of balsamic glaze before serving.
- These can be made ahead and stored in the fridge for up to 24 hours.

N.V.: Calories: 120, Fat: 9g, Carbs: 6g, Protein: 4g, Sugar: 4g, Sodium: 140 mg, Potassium: 200 mg, Cholesterol: 10 mg

PROSCIUTTO-WRAPPED ASPARAGUS

PREPARATION TIME: 10 min
COOKING TIME: 10 min
MODE OF COOKING: Baking
SERVINGS: 4
INGREDIENTS:

- 12 asparagus spears, trimmed
- 6 slices prosciutto, halved lengthwise
- 1 Tbsp olive oil
- 1 tsp lemon juice
- Salt and pepper to taste

DIRECTIONS:

1. Preheat oven to 400°F (204°C).
2. Wrap each asparagus spear with a half slice of prosciutto.
3. Place the wrapped asparagus on a baking sheet and drizzle with olive oil, lemon juice, salt, and pepper.
4. Bake for 10 minutes, until the prosciutto is crispy and the asparagus is tender.

TIPS:

- Serve with a side of lemon wedges for extra zing.
- For a different twist, try wrapping the asparagus with thin slices of smoked salmon.

N.V.: Calories: 80, Fat: 6g, Carbs: 2g, Protein: 6g, Sugar: 0g, Sodium: 220 mg, Potassium: 200 mg, Cholesterol: 15 mg

CUCUMBER CANAPÉS WITH SMOKED SALMON

PREPARATION TIME: 10 min
COOKING TIME: None
MODE OF COOKING: No Cooking
SERVINGS: 4
INGREDIENTS:

- 1 large cucumber, sliced into rounds
- 4 oz smoked salmon, thinly sliced
- 4 Tbsp lactose-free cream cheese
- 1 Tbsp fresh dill, chopped
- 1 tsp lemon zest
- Salt and pepper to taste

DIRECTIONS:

1. Spread a thin layer of lactose-free cream cheese on each cucumber slice.
2. Top with a small piece of smoked salmon.
3. Sprinkle with fresh dill, lemon zest, salt, and pepper.

TIPS:

- Add a caper or two on top for a burst of briny flavor.
- Serve immediately for the best texture.

N.V.: Calories: 90, Fat: 7g, Carbs: 3g, Protein: 5g, Sugar: 2g, Sodium: 180 mg, Potassium: 150 mg, Cholesterol: 15 mg

BAKED ZUCCHINI FRIES WITH PARMESAN

PREPARATION TIME: 10 min
COOKING TIME: 20 min
MODE OF COOKING: Baking
SERVINGS: 4
INGREDIENTS:

- 2 medium zucchinis, cut into sticks
- 1/2 cup gluten-free breadcrumbs
- 1/4 cup lactose-free Parmesan cheese, grated
- 1 tsp dried oregano
- 1 egg, beaten
- 1 Tbsp olive oil
- Salt and pepper to taste

DIRECTIONS:

1. Preheat oven to 425°F (218°C).
2. In a bowl, mix gluten-free breadcrumbs, Parmesan cheese, oregano, salt, and pepper.
3. Dip each zucchini stick into the beaten egg, then coat with the breadcrumb mixture.
4. Place the zucchini sticks on a baking sheet lined with parchment paper.
5. Drizzle with olive oil and bake for 20 minutes until golden and crispy.

TIPS:

- Serve with a side of marinara sauce for dipping.
- For extra crunch, use panko-style gluten-free breadcrumbs.

N.V.: Calories: 150, Fat: 8g, Carbs: 14g, Protein: 6g, Sugar: 3g, Sodium: 220 mg, Potassium: 300 mg, Cholesterol: 55 mg

CAPRESE SKEWERS WITH BALSAMIC GLAZE

PREPARATION TIME: 10 min
COOKING TIME: None
MODE OF COOKING: No Cooking
SERVINGS: 4
INGREDIENTS:

- 12 cherry tomatoes
- 12 small fresh mozzarella balls (lactose-free)
- 12 fresh basil leaves
- 2 Tbsp balsamic glaze
- 1 Tbsp olive oil
- Salt and pepper to taste

DIRECTIONS:

1. Thread one cherry tomato, one mozzarella ball, and one basil leaf onto each skewer.
2. Arrange the skewers on a serving platter.
3. Drizzle with balsamic glaze and olive oil, and season with salt and pepper.

TIPS:

- For a burst of flavor, marinate the mozzarella balls in olive oil and herbs before assembling.
- These can be made ahead and refrigerated until ready to serve.

N.V.: Calories: 110, Fat: 8g, Carbs: 5g, Protein: 5g, Sugar: 4g, Sodium: 120 mg, Potassium: 150 mg, Cholesterol: 10 mg

SHRIMP COCKTAIL WITH LEMON-HERB DIP

PREPARATION TIME: 10 min
COOKING TIME: 5 min
MODE OF COOKING: Stovetop
SERVINGS: 4
INGREDIENTS:

- 1 lb. large shrimp, peeled and deveined
- 1 lemon, juiced
- 2 Tbsp fresh parsley, chopped
- 1 Tbsp fresh dill, chopped
- 1/4 cup lactose-free Greek yogurt

- 1 Tbsp Dijon mustard
- Salt and pepper to taste

DIRECTIONS:

1. Bring a pot of water to a boil, then add the shrimp and cook for 3-4 minutes until they turn pink and opaque. Drain and cool.
2. In a small bowl, mix the Greek yogurt, Dijon mustard, lemon juice, parsley, dill, salt, and pepper to make the dip.
3. Arrange the shrimp on a serving platter and serve with the lemon-herb dip.

TIPS:

- Garnish the shrimp with additional lemon wedges for extra zing.
- For a spicier dip, add a pinch of cayenne pepper.

N.V.: Calories: 130, Fat: 3g, Carbs: 5g, Protein: 22g, Sugar: 2g, Sodium: 220 mg, Potassium: 250 mg, Cholesterol: 170 mg

STUFFED CUCUMBER BITES

PREPARATION TIME: 10 min
COOKING TIME: None
MODE OF COOKING: No Cooking
SERVINGS: 4
INGREDIENTS:

- 1 large cucumber, cut into thick slices
- 1/2 cup lactose-free cream cheese
- 1/4 cup lactose-free feta cheese, crumbled
- 1 Tbsp fresh dill, chopped
- 1 Tbsp lemon juice
- Salt and pepper to taste

DIRECTIONS:

1. Using a small spoon, scoop out the center of each cucumber slice to create a well, leaving the bottom intact.
2. In a bowl, mix lactose-free cream cheese, feta cheese, dill, lemon juice, salt, and pepper until well combined.
3. Spoon the cheese mixture into each cucumber slice.
4. Arrange on a platter and serve chilled.

TIPS:

- Garnish with extra dill or a sprinkle of paprika for added color.
- These can be made ahead and stored in the fridge until ready to serve.

N.V.: Calories: 80, Fat: 6g, Carbs: 3g, Protein: 3g, Sugar: 2g, Sodium: 140 mg, Potassium: 150 mg, Cholesterol: 15 mg

SMOKED SALMON CUCUMBER BITES

PREPARATION TIME: 10 min
COOKING TIME: None
MODE OF COOKING: No Cooking
SERVINGS: 4
INGREDIENTS:

- 1 large cucumber, sliced into rounds
- 4 oz smoked salmon, sliced
- 2 Tbsp lactose-free cream cheese
- 1 tsp lemon zest
- Fresh dill for garnish
- Salt and pepper to taste

DIRECTIONS:

1. Spread a small amount of lactose-free cream cheese on each cucumber round.
2. Top with a slice of smoked salmon.
3. Sprinkle with lemon zest, salt, and pepper.
4. Garnish with fresh dill.

TIPS:

- Serve immediately for the best texture.
- Add a caper on top of each bite for an extra burst of flavor.

N.V.: Calories: 90, Fat: 5g, Carbs: 3g, Protein: 8g, Sugar: 1g, Sodium: 240 mg, Potassium: 150 mg, Cholesterol: 20 mg

POLENTA BITES WITH ROASTED RED PEPPER

PREPARATION TIME: 10 min
COOKING TIME: 20 min
MODE OF COOKING: Baking
SERVINGS: 4
INGREDIENTS:

- 1 tube of pre-cooked polenta, sliced into rounds

- 1/2 cup roasted red peppers, sliced
- 1/4 cup lactose-free feta cheese, crumbled
- 1 Tbsp olive oil
- 1 tsp dried oregano
- Salt and pepper to taste

DIRECTIONS:
1. Preheat oven to 375°F (190°C).
2. Place the polenta rounds on a baking sheet lined with parchment paper.
3. Drizzle with olive oil and season with salt, pepper, and oregano.
4. Bake for 15 minutes, until the edges are crispy.
5. Top each polenta round with a slice of roasted red pepper and a sprinkle of feta cheese.
6. Return to the oven for an additional 5 minutes to warm the toppings.

TIPS:
- These bites are best served warm, straight from the oven.
- Garnish with fresh basil for an extra touch of flavor.

N.V.: Calories: 120, Fat: 6g, Carbs: 14g, Protein: 3g, Sugar: 1g, Sodium: 200 mg, Potassium: 150 mg, Cholesterol: 10 mg

ROASTED CARROT AND ZUCCHINI STICKS

PREPARATION TIME: 10 min
COOKING TIME: 20 min
MODE OF COOKING: Roasting
SERVINGS: 4
INGREDIENTS:
- 2 large carrots, cut into sticks
- 2 medium zucchinis, cut into sticks
- 2 Tbsp olive oil
- 1 tsp smoked paprika
- 1/2 tsp ground cumin
- Salt and pepper to taste

DIRECTIONS:
1. Preheat oven to 400°F (204°C).
2. Toss the carrot and zucchini sticks with olive oil, smoked paprika, cumin, salt, and pepper.
3. Spread the vegetables in a single layer on a baking sheet.
4. Roast for 20 minutes, turning halfway through, until the vegetables are tender and slightly caramelized.

TIPS:
- Serve with a side of low-FODMAP hummus or yogurt dip.
- For extra crispiness, broil the vegetables for the last 2-3 minutes.

N.V.: Calories: 110, Fat: 7g, Carbs: 10g, Protein: 2g, Sugar: 4g, Sodium: 120 mg, Potassium: 450 mg, Cholesterol: 0 mg

SWEET POTATO CROSTINI WITH AVOCADO AND POMEGRANATE

PREPARATION TIME: 10 min
COOKING TIME: 20 min
MODE OF COOKING: Baking
SERVINGS: 4
INGREDIENTS:
- 1 large sweet potato, sliced into rounds
- 1 ripe avocado, mashed
- 1/4 cup pomegranate seeds
- 1 Tbsp olive oil
- 1 tsp lime juice
- Salt and pepper to taste
- Fresh cilantro for garnish

DIRECTIONS:
1. Preheat oven to 400°F (204°C).
2. Toss the sweet potato rounds with olive oil, salt, and pepper.
3. Arrange the rounds on a baking sheet and bake for 15-20 minutes, until tender and slightly crispy.
4. Top each sweet potato round with a dollop of mashed avocado, pomegranate seeds, and a sprinkle of lime juice.
5. Garnish with fresh cilantro before serving.

TIPS:
- These crostini are best served immediately while the sweet potatoes are warm.

- Add a pinch of red pepper flakes for a spicy kick.

N.V.: Calories: 180, Fat: 9g, Carbs: 24g, Protein: 2g, Sugar: 6g, Sodium: 100 mg, Potassium: 450 mg, Cholesterol: 0 mg

BAKED POLENTA BITES WITH TOMATO AND BASIL

PREPARATION TIME: 10 min
COOKING TIME: 20 min
MODE OF COOKING: Baking
SERVINGS: 4
INGREDIENTS:
- 1 tube of pre-cooked polenta, sliced into rounds
- 1/2 cup cherry tomatoes, halved
- 1/4 cup lactose-free mozzarella cheese, shredded
- 2 Tbsp fresh basil, chopped
- 1 Tbsp olive oil
- Salt and pepper to taste

DIRECTIONS:
1. Preheat oven to 375°F (190°C).
2. Arrange the polenta rounds on a baking sheet lined with parchment paper.
3. Top each polenta round with a few cherry tomato halves and a sprinkle of mozzarella cheese.
4. Drizzle with olive oil and season with salt and pepper.
5. Bake for 15-20 minutes, until the cheese is melted and the polenta is crispy around the edges.
6. Garnish with fresh basil before serving.

TIPS:
- These bites are perfect for parties and can be served warm or at room temperature.
- Add a drizzle of balsamic glaze for extra flavor.

N.V.: Calories: 130, Fat: 7g, Carbs: 14g, Protein: 4g, Sugar: 2g, Sodium: 180 mg, Potassium: 150 mg, Cholesterol: 10 mg

CHAPTER 10: DESSERT DELIGHTS

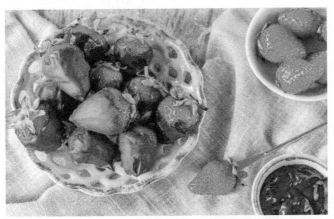

Navigating a low-FODMAP diet often feels like wandering a narrow pathway flanked by vast plains of dietary restrictions. Yet, as we've explored various meal options in this cookbook, maintaining a rich and fulfilling diet is very much within reach. This becomes even more delightful when we reach the realm of desserts where indulgence meets ingenuity. Desserts often conjure images of decadent chocolate, creamy pastries, and sugary confections foods that typically sit on the "avoid" list of a low-FODMAP diet. However, the joy of dessert doesn't have to be lost. Imagine reinventing these treats in a way that not only respects your dietary needs but also elevates your dining experience to exciting new heights. In this chapter, we dive into that delicious endeavor.

The fear of missing out, especially when it comes to sweet treats, is very real. But what if I told you that with a few clever adjustments, you can enjoy sumptuous desserts that are both gut-friendly and crowd-pleasers? Our sensory exploration does not end at the dinner table. It extends to a world where fruit-based favorites soothe the palate, where light, fluffy desserts dance in our mouths, and indulgent yet safe sweets cater to our deepest cravings. One of the crowning glories of mastering the low-FODMAP diet is the ability to turn potential dietary limitations into a challenge for your culinary creativity. From fruit tarts that utilize seasonal berries to velvety mousses with acceptable alternatives to conventional sweeteners, every recipe in this chapter has been designed to ensure you can end every meal on a sweet note without discomfort. Moreover, these desserts are not just about adhering to dietary restrictions; they are about celebrating food and reclaiming the joy of eating in every spoonful. As we progress, remember that each treat you master is a step towards better managing digestive health, while still allowing yourself the pleasure of good, earnest cooking. Let's whisk away the notion that desserts are off-limits, and instead, dive into devising treats that delight both the palate and the gut. Here's to a sweet finish with no regrets!

DECADENT CHOCOLATE AVOCADO MOUSSE

PREPARATION TIME: 10 min
COOKING TIME: None
MODE OF COOKING: No Cooking
SERVINGS: 4
INGREDIENTS:

- 2 ripe avocados
- 1/4 cup unsweetened cocoa powder
- 1/4 cup maple syrup
- 1/4 cup almond milk (unsweetened)
- 1 tsp vanilla extract
- Pinch of salt
- Fresh berries for garnish (optional)

DIRECTIONS:

1. In a blender or food processor, combine avocados, cocoa powder, maple syrup, almond milk, vanilla extract, and a pinch of salt.
2. Blend until smooth and creamy.
3. Spoon the mousse into serving bowls and refrigerate for at least 30 minutes to set.
4. Garnish with fresh berries if desired before serving.

TIPS:

- Add a pinch of cinnamon or chili powder for a unique flavor twist.
- This mousse can be stored in the fridge for up to 2 days.

N.V.: Calories: 240, Fat: 18g, Carbs: 22g, Protein: 3g, Sugar: 12g, Sodium: 40 mg, Potassium: 500 mg, Cholesterol: 0 mg

RASPBERRY COCONUT MACAROONS

PREPARATION TIME: 10 min
COOKING TIME: 20 min
MODE OF COOKING: Baking
SERVINGS: 12
INGREDIENTS:

- 2 cups unsweetened shredded coconut
- 1/4 cup almond flour
- 1/4 cup maple syrup
- 1/4 cup fresh raspberries, mashed
- 1 tsp vanilla extract
- Pinch of salt

DIRECTIONS:

1. Preheat oven to 325°F (160°C). Line a baking sheet with parchment paper.
2. In a large bowl, combine shredded coconut, almond flour, maple syrup, mashed raspberries, vanilla extract, and salt.
3. Mix until all ingredients are well combined.
4. Scoop tablespoon-sized mounds of the mixture onto the prepared baking sheet.
5. Bake for 18-20 minutes, or until the edges are golden brown.
6. Let cool completely before serving.

TIPS:

- Drizzle with melted dark chocolate for an extra indulgence.
- Store in an airtight container for up to 5 days.

N.V.: Calories: 100, Fat: 7g, Carbs: 9g, Protein: 2g, Sugar: 6g, Sodium: 40 mg, Potassium: 100 mg, Cholesterol: 0 mg

CHOCOLATE-DIPPED STRAWBERRIES

PREPARATION TIME: 5 min
COOKING TIME: 5 min
MODE OF COOKING: Stovetop
SERVINGS: 4
INGREDIENTS:

- 1 cup fresh strawberries
- 1/2 cup dairy-free dark chocolate chips
- 1 tsp coconut oil

DIRECTIONS:

1. Wash and thoroughly dry the strawberries.
2. In a small saucepan, melt the dark chocolate chips and coconut oil over low heat, stirring until smooth.
3. Dip each strawberry into the melted chocolate, covering about two-thirds of the berry.
4. Place the chocolate-dipped strawberries on a parchment-lined

baking sheet and refrigerate for 15 minutes, or until the chocolate is set.

TIPS:

- Sprinkle with crushed nuts or shredded coconut before the chocolate sets for extra texture.
- Serve chilled for a refreshing dessert or snack.

N.V.: Calories: 120, Fat: 8g, Carbs: 14g, Protein: 1g, Sugar: 9g, Sodium: 0 mg, Potassium: 150 mg, Cholesterol: 0 mg

PEANUT BUTTER CHOCOLATE CHIP COOKIES

PREPARATION TIME: 10 min
COOKING TIME: 12 min
MODE OF COOKING: Baking
SERVINGS: 12 cookies
INGREDIENTS:

- 1 cup natural peanut butter
- 1/2 cup coconut sugar
- 1 egg (or flax egg for vegan option)
- 1/2 tsp baking soda
- 1/2 cup dairy-free chocolate chips

DIRECTIONS:

1. Preheat oven to 350°F (175°C). Line a baking sheet with parchment paper.
2. In a bowl, mix peanut butter, coconut sugar, egg, and baking soda until well combined.
3. Fold in the chocolate chips.
4. Scoop tablespoon-sized balls of dough onto the prepared baking sheet and flatten slightly with a fork.
5. Bake for 10-12 minutes, or until the edges are golden. Let cool on the baking sheet for 5 minutes before transferring to a wire rack to cool completely.

TIPS:

- Add a sprinkle of sea salt on top of the cookies before baking for a sweet-salty flavor.
- Store in an airtight container for up to a week.

N.V.: Calories: 190, Fat: 14g, Carbs: 14g, Protein: 5g, Sugar: 9g, Sodium: 100 mg, Potassium: 200 mg, Cholesterol: 20 mg

CHOCOLATE COCONUT MACAROONS

PREPARATION TIME: 10 min
COOKING TIME: 15 min
MODE OF COOKING: Baking
SERVINGS: 12
INGREDIENTS:

- 2 cups unsweetened shredded coconut
- 1/2 cup almond flour
- 1/4 cup maple syrup
- 1/4 cup coconut oil, melted
- 1/2 cup dairy-free dark chocolate chips
- 1 tsp vanilla extract
- Pinch of salt

DIRECTIONS:

1. Preheat oven to 325°F (160°C). Line a baking sheet with parchment paper.
2. In a large bowl, mix shredded coconut, almond flour, maple syrup, melted coconut oil, vanilla extract, and salt until well combined.
3. Scoop tablespoon-sized mounds of the mixture onto the prepared baking sheet.
4. Bake for 12-15 minutes, or until the edges are golden brown.
5. In a small saucepan, melt the dark chocolate chips over low heat, stirring until smooth.
6. Drizzle the melted chocolate over the macaroons or dip the bottoms into the chocolate.

TIPS:

- Store in an airtight container for up to a week.
- For an extra indulgent treat, sprinkle the macaroons with sea salt before the chocolate sets.

N.V.: Calories: 140, Fat: 12g, Carbs: 10g, Protein: 2g, Sugar: 7g, Sodium: 30 mg, Potassium: 120 mg, Cholesterol: 0 mg

LEMON POPPY SEED MUFFINS

PREPARATION TIME: 10 min
COOKING TIME: 20 min
MODE OF COOKING: Baking
SERVINGS: 8
INGREDIENTS:

- 1 1/2 cups almond flour
- 1/4 cup coconut sugar
- 2 Tbsp poppy seeds
- 1/4 cup coconut oil, melted
- 3 large eggs
- 1/4 cup almond milk (unsweetened)
- 2 Tbsp lemon juice
- 1 Tbsp lemon zest
- 1 tsp baking powder
- 1/2 tsp vanilla extract
- Pinch of salt

DIRECTIONS:

1. Preheat oven to 350°F (175°C). Line a muffin tin with paper liners.
2. In a large bowl, whisk together almond flour, coconut sugar, poppy seeds, baking powder, and salt.
3. In another bowl, mix melted coconut oil, eggs, almond milk, lemon juice, lemon zest, and vanilla extract until well combined.
4. Add the wet ingredients to the dry ingredients and stir until just combined.
5. Divide the batter evenly among the muffin cups.
6. Bake for 18-20 minutes, or until a toothpick inserted into the center comes out clean.
7. Let the muffins cool in the tin for 5 minutes, then transfer to a wire rack to cool completely.

TIPS:

- Drizzle with a simple lemon glaze made from lemon juice and powdered sugar for extra sweetness.
- Store muffins in an airtight container at room temperature for up to 3 days.

N.V.: Calories: 180, Fat: 14g, Carbs: 10g, Protein: 5g, Sugar: 5g, Sodium: 100 mg, Potassium: 150 mg, Cholesterol: 55 mg

VANILLA SOUFFLÉ

PREPARATION TIME: 15 min
COOKING TIME: 15 min
MODE OF COOKING: Baking
SERVINGS: 4
INGREDIENTS:

- 3 large eggs, separated
- 1/4 cup almond milk (unsweetened)
- 2 Tbsp coconut sugar
- 1 Tbsp gluten-free flour
- 1 tsp vanilla extract
- Pinch of salt
- Powdered sugar for dusting (optional)

DIRECTIONS:

1. Preheat oven to 375°F (190°C). Grease four ramekins with coconut oil and dust with a little gluten-free flour.
2. In a small saucepan, whisk together almond milk, coconut sugar, gluten-free flour, and salt over medium heat until thickened, about 2 minutes. Remove from heat and stir in vanilla extract.
3. In a separate bowl, whisk the egg yolks, then slowly add the warm milk mixture, stirring constantly.
4. In another bowl, beat the egg whites until stiff peaks form.
5. Gently fold the egg whites into the yolk mixture until fully combined.
6. Spoon the mixture into the prepared ramekins and smooth the tops.
7. Bake for 15 minutes, or until the soufflés are puffed and golden.
8. Dust with powdered sugar before serving if desired.

TIPS:

- Serve immediately as soufflés will deflate quickly.
- Add a dollop of whipped coconut cream for an extra treat.

N.V.: Calories: 130, Fat: 6g, Carbs: 10g, Protein: 7g, Sugar: 6g, Sodium: 60 mg, Potassium: 70 mg, Cholesterol: 140 mg

FLUFFY COCONUT RICE PUDDING

PREPARATION TIME: 5 min
COOKING TIME: 25 min
MODE OF COOKING: Stovetop
SERVINGS: 4
INGREDIENTS:

- 1/2 cup jasmine rice
- 1 1/2 cups coconut milk (full fat)
- 1/4 cup coconut sugar
- 1 tsp vanilla extract
- 1/4 tsp ground cinnamon
- Fresh fruit for topping (optional)

DIRECTIONS:

1. In a medium saucepan, combine jasmine rice, coconut milk, coconut sugar, and cinnamon.
2. Bring to a simmer over medium heat, stirring occasionally.
3. Reduce heat to low, cover, and cook for 20-25 minutes, or until the rice is tender and the mixture is creamy.
4. Remove from heat and stir in vanilla extract.
5. Spoon the rice pudding into serving bowls and top with fresh fruit if desired.

TIPS:

- Serve warm or chilled, depending on your preference.
- Sprinkle with toasted coconut flakes for added texture.

N.V.: Calories: 180, Fat: 10g, Carbs: 20g, Protein: 2g, Sugar: 8g, Sodium: 30 mg, Potassium: 200 mg, Cholesterol: 0 mg

STRAWBERRY YOGURT PARFAIT

PREPARATION TIME: 5 min
COOKING TIME: None
MODE OF COOKING: No Cooking
SERVINGS: 2
INGREDIENTS:

- 1 cup lactose-free Greek yogurt
- 1/2 cup fresh strawberries, sliced
- 1/4 cup gluten-free granola
- 1 Tbsp maple syrup
- 1 tsp chia seeds (optional)

DIRECTIONS:

1. In two serving glasses, layer half of the Greek yogurt.
2. Add a layer of sliced strawberries and drizzle with a little maple syrup.
3. Sprinkle with granola and chia seeds if using.
4. Repeat the layers with the remaining ingredients.

TIPS:

- Add other low-FODMAP fruits like blueberries or bananas for variety.
- Serve immediately to keep the granola crunchy.

N.V.: Calories: 180, Fat: 6g, Carbs: 22g, Protein: 10g, Sugar: 12g, Sodium: 60 mg, Potassium: 200 mg, Cholesterol: 10 mg

ALMOND FLOUR LEMON COOKIES

PREPARATION TIME: 10 min
COOKING TIME: 12 min
MODE OF COOKING: Baking
SERVINGS: 12 cookies
INGREDIENTS:

- 1 1/2 cups almond flour
- 1/4 cup coconut sugar
- 1/4 cup coconut oil, melted
- 1 Tbsp lemon juice
- 1 Tbsp lemon zest
- 1 tsp vanilla extract
- 1/2 tsp baking powder
- Pinch of salt

DIRECTIONS:

1. Preheat oven to 350°F (175°C). Line a baking sheet with parchment paper.
2. In a bowl, mix almond flour, coconut sugar, baking powder, and salt.
3. Add melted coconut oil, lemon juice, lemon zest, and vanilla extract to the dry ingredients and stir until a dough forms.

4. Scoop tablespoon-sized balls of dough onto the prepared baking sheet and flatten slightly.
5. Bake for 10-12 minutes, or until the edges are golden.
6. Let cool on the baking sheet for 5 minutes before transferring to a wire rack to cool completely.

TIPS:
- Store cookies in an airtight container at room temperature for up to 5 days.
- For an extra burst of lemon flavor, drizzle with a simple lemon glaze made from powdered sugar and lemon juice.

N.V.: Calories: 110, Fat: 8g, Carbs: 8g, Protein: 2g, Sugar: 5g, Sodium: 40 mg, Potassium: 40 mg, Cholesterol: 0 mg

FLUFFY COCONUT PANCAKES

PREPARATION TIME: 5 min
COOKING TIME: 10 min
MODE OF COOKING: Stovetop
SERVINGS: 4
INGREDIENTS:
- 1 cup coconut flour
- 1/4 cup tapioca flour
- 1 Tbsp coconut sugar
- 1 tsp baking powder
- 1/4 tsp salt
- 3 large eggs
- 1 cup almond milk (unsweetened)
- 1 tsp vanilla extract
- Coconut oil for cooking

DIRECTIONS:
1. In a bowl, whisk together coconut flour, tapioca flour, coconut sugar, baking powder, and salt.
2. In another bowl, beat eggs, almond milk, and vanilla extract until smooth.
3. Combine the wet and dry ingredients, stirring until just combined.
4. Heat a skillet over medium heat and grease with coconut oil.
5. Pour 1/4 cup of batter onto the skillet for each pancake.

6. Cook for 2-3 minutes, or until bubbles form on the surface, then flip and cook for another 2 minutes until golden brown.

TIPS:
- Serve with fresh fruit, a drizzle of maple syrup, or a dollop of coconut whipped cream.
- For extra fluffiness, let the batter rest for a few minutes before cooking.

N.V.: Calories: 180, Fat: 11g, Carbs: 12g, Protein: 5g, Sugar: 3g, Sodium: 150 mg, Potassium: 100 mg, Cholesterol: 100 mg

LEMON RICOTTA PANCAKES

PREPARATION TIME: 10 min
COOKING TIME: 10 min
MODE OF COOKING: Stovetop
SERVINGS: 4
INGREDIENTS:
- 1 cup almond flour
- 1/2 cup lactose-free ricotta cheese
- 2 large eggs
- 1/4 cup almond milk (unsweetened)
- 2 Tbsp lemon juice
- 1 Tbsp lemon zest
- 1 Tbsp maple syrup
- 1 tsp vanilla extract
- 1/2 tsp baking powder
- Pinch of salt
- Coconut oil for cooking

DIRECTIONS:
1. In a large bowl, whisk together almond flour, baking powder, and salt.
2. In another bowl, mix ricotta cheese, eggs, almond milk, lemon juice, lemon zest, maple syrup, and vanilla extract until smooth.
3. Combine the wet and dry ingredients, stirring until just incorporated.
4. Heat a skillet over medium heat and lightly grease with coconut oil.
5. Pour 1/4 cup of batter onto the skillet for each pancake.
6. Cook for 2-3 minutes, or until bubbles form on the surface, then flip and cook

for another 2 minutes until golden brown.

TIPS:
- Serve with fresh berries and a drizzle of maple syrup for extra flavor.
- These pancakes can be made ahead and reheated in a toaster or oven.

N.V.: Calories: 160, Fat: 11g, Carbs: 10g, Protein: 7g, Sugar: 4g, Sodium: 130 mg, Potassium: 100 mg, Cholesterol: 80 mg

GRILLED PINEAPPLE WITH LIME AND MINT

PREPARATION TIME: 10 min
COOKING TIME: 10 min
MODE OF COOKING: Grilling
SERVINGS: 4
INGREDIENTS:
- 1 pineapple, peeled, cored, and sliced into rings
- 2 Tbsp lime juice
- 1 Tbsp maple syrup
- 1 Tbsp fresh mint, chopped
- 1 tsp lime zest

DIRECTIONS:
1. Preheat grill to medium-high heat.
2. In a small bowl, mix lime juice, maple syrup, and lime zest.
3. Brush the pineapple slices with the lime mixture.
4. Grill the pineapple for 3-4 minutes on each side, until caramelized and tender.
5. Remove from the grill and sprinkle with fresh mint.

TIPS:
- Serve with a dollop of coconut yogurt for a refreshing contrast.
- For a spicy twist, add a pinch of chili powder to the lime mixture.

N.V.: Calories: 90, Fat: 0g, Carbs: 23g, Protein: 1g, Sugar: 18g, Sodium: 2 mg, Potassium: 200 mg, Cholesterol: 0 mg

BAKED PEACHES WITH CINNAMON ALMOND CRUMBLE

PREPARATION TIME: 10 min
COOKING TIME: 20 min
MODE OF COOKING: Baking
SERVINGS: 4
INGREDIENTS:
- 4 ripe peaches, halved and pitted
- 1/4 cup almond flour
- 2 Tbsp gluten-free oats
- 2 Tbsp coconut sugar
- 2 Tbsp coconut oil, melted
- 1 tsp ground cinnamon
- 1/4 tsp vanilla extract

DIRECTIONS:
1. Preheat oven to 350°F (175°C).
2. In a small bowl, mix almond flour, oats, coconut sugar, melted coconut oil, cinnamon, and vanilla extract until crumbly.
3. Place peach halves in a baking dish, cut side up.
4. Spoon the crumble mixture onto the peaches, pressing it down slightly.
5. Bake for 20 minutes, or until the peaches are tender and the crumble is golden.

TIPS:
- Serve with a scoop of dairy-free vanilla ice cream or a dollop of coconut cream.
- For a nut-free option, replace almond flour with additional oats.

N.V.: Calories: 160, Fat: 9g, Carbs: 20g, Protein: 2g, Sugar: 15g, Sodium: 5 mg, Potassium: 200 mg, Cholesterol: 0 mg

GRILLED BANANA BOATS

PREPARATION TIME: 5 min
COOKING TIME: 10 min
MODE OF COOKING: Grilling
SERVINGS: 4
INGREDIENTS:

- 4 bananas, unpeeled, ends trimmed
- 1/4 cup dairy-free dark chocolate chips
- 1/4 cup chopped walnuts
- 2 Tbsp shredded coconut
- 1 tsp cinnamon

DIRECTIONS:

1. Preheat grill to medium heat.
2. Slice each banana lengthwise down the middle, being careful not to cut through the bottom peel.
3. Gently open the bananas and stuff with chocolate chips, walnuts, shredded coconut, and a sprinkle of cinnamon.
4. Wrap each banana in aluminum foil and place on the grill.
5. Grill for 8-10 minutes, or until the bananas are soft and the chocolate is melted.
6. Carefully unwrap and serve immediately.

TIPS:

- Top with a dollop of dairy-free whipped cream or a scoop of vanilla coconut ice cream.
- For a nut-free version, replace walnuts with sunflower seeds.

N.V.: Calories: 180, Fat: 9g, Carbs: 25g, Protein: 3g, Sugar: 15g, Sodium: 2 mg, Potassium: 350 mg, Cholesterol: 0 mg

BLUEBERRY LEMON PARFAIT

PREPARATION TIME: 10 min
COOKING TIME: None
MODE OF COOKING: No Cooking
SERVINGS: 4
INGREDIENTS:

- 1 cup lactose-free Greek yogurt
- 1 cup fresh blueberries
- 2 Tbsp lemon juice
- 1 Tbsp maple syrup
- 1/2 cup gluten-free granola
- 1 tsp lemon zest

DIRECTIONS:

1. In a small bowl, mix the lactose-free Greek yogurt with lemon juice, lemon zest, and maple syrup.
2. In serving glasses, layer the yogurt mixture with fresh blueberries and gluten-free granola.
3. Top with a few extra blueberries and a sprinkle of lemon zest.

TIPS:

- For added flavor, mix in a few fresh mint leaves with the blueberries.
- Serve immediately to keep the granola crunchy.

N.V.: Calories: 160, Fat: 4g, Carbs: 27g, Protein: 6g, Sugar: 16g, Sodium: 50 mg, Potassium: 200 mg, Cholesterol: 5 mg

TROPICAL FRUIT SALAD WITH LIME DRESSING

PREPARATION TIME: 10 min
COOKING TIME: None
MODE OF COOKING: No Cooking
SERVINGS: 4
INGREDIENTS:

- 1 ripe mango, diced
- 1 cup pineapple chunks
- 1 kiwi, peeled and sliced
- 1/2 cup diced papaya
- 1/4 cup shredded coconut
- 2 Tbsp lime juice
- 1 Tbsp honey (use maple syrup for vegan option)
- 1 Tbsp fresh mint, chopped

DIRECTIONS:

1. In a large bowl, combine mango, pineapple, kiwi, and papaya.
2. In a small bowl, whisk together lime juice, honey, and fresh mint.
3. Drizzle the lime dressing over the fruit and toss gently to combine.

4. Sprinkle with shredded coconut before serving.

TIPS:
- Serve chilled for a refreshing treat on a hot day.
- Add a handful of pomegranate seeds for extra color and flavor.

N.V.: Calories: 120, Fat: 3g, Carbs: 26g, Protein: 1g, Sugar: 20g, Sodium: 10 mg, Potassium: 250 mg, Cholesterol: 0 mg

GRILLED PEACHES WITH BALSAMIC GLAZE

PREPARATION TIME: 5 min
COOKING TIME: 10 min
MODE OF COOKING: Grilling
SERVINGS: 4
INGREDIENTS:
- 4 ripe peaches, halved and pitted
- 1/4 cup balsamic vinegar
- 2 Tbsp maple syrup
- 1 tsp fresh rosemary, chopped (optional)
- 1/4 cup chopped pistachios

DIRECTIONS:
1. Preheat grill to medium-high heat.
2. In a small saucepan, combine balsamic vinegar, maple syrup, and rosemary (if using). Bring to a simmer over medium heat and cook until reduced by half, about 5 minutes.
3. Brush the peach halves with a little of the balsamic glaze.
4. Grill the peaches, cut side down, for 4-5 minutes, or until grill marks appear and the peaches are slightly softened.
5. Remove from the grill and drizzle with the remaining balsamic glaze.
6. Sprinkle with chopped pistachios before serving.

TIPS:
- Serve with a dollop of dairy-free whipped cream or yogurt.
- For a sweeter variation, add a sprinkle of cinnamon to the peaches before grilling.

N.V.: Calories: 130, Fat: 4g, Carbs: 23g, Protein: 2g, Sugar: 18g, Sodium: 5 mg, Potassium: 250 mg, Cholesterol: 0 mg

CHAPTER 11: BOOSTING FLAVORS

Imagine you're about to savor a beautifully prepared meal, and just as you're ready to dive in, you realize it needs a little something extra. This is where the magic of flavor enhancement truly shines, transforming the ordinary into the extraordinary. In the world of a low-FODMAP diet, where the usual suspects like onion and garlic are off the menu, crafting mouthwatering dishes with depth can seem like a culinary conundrum. But fret not! This chapter is dedicated to elevating your cooking without the FODMAP fuss, using ingredients that soothe rather than upset your system.

Flavors are the soul of our meals; they can transport us to different places and conjure memories both sweet and savory. Learning how to enhance flavors while adhering to a low-FODMAP diet means you won't have to sacrifice satisfaction for comfort. Think of it as your toolkit for infusing richness into every dish, whether it's a zesty dressing, a robust sauce, or a custom spice blend.

Let's begin with home-made condiments. The joy of mixing up your own ketchup without the high-fructose corn syrup, or whisking together a mustard that's just the right blend of tangy and spicy, can be both rewarding and reassuring. You know exactly what goes into it, ensuring that you keep within safe eating boundaries while still tickling your taste buds. Next, we wade into the aromatic world of sauces. Imagine drizzling a ginger-infused glaze over a grilled chicken or swirling a basil-rich pesto through your pasta. These sauces don't just add moisture; they layer flavors, creating more nuanced, satisfying bites.

Finally, let's not underestimate the power of spice blends. With the right combination of herbs and spices, even a simple roasted vegetable can become the highlight of your meal. Crafting your blend means you have control that sprinkle of cinnamon or that dash of thyme is not just adding flavor, but also ensuring that you stay well within your dietary comfort zone.

By the end of this chapter, you'll be ready to add that "little something extra" to every meal, ensuring your culinary creations are both delicious and digestion-friendly.

CLASSIC BALSAMIC VINAIGRETTE

PREPARATION TIME: 5 min
COOKING TIME: None
MODE OF COOKING: No Cooking
SERVINGS: 8 (2 Tbsp per serving)
INGREDIENTS:

- 1/2 cup extra-virgin olive oil
- 1/4 cup balsamic vinegar
- 1 tsp Dijon mustard
- 1 tsp maple syrup
- 1/2 tsp salt
- 1/4 tsp black pepper

DIRECTIONS:

1. In a small bowl, whisk together balsamic vinegar, Dijon mustard, maple syrup, salt, and black pepper.
2. Slowly drizzle in the olive oil while whisking continuously until the mixture is emulsified.
3. Adjust seasoning to taste and serve over salads or roasted vegetables.

TIPS:

- Store in a sealed container in the refrigerator for up to a week.
- Shake well before each use if the dressing separates.

N.V.: Calories: 100, Fat: 10g, Carbs: 2g, Protein: 0g, Sugar: 1g, Sodium: 150 mg, Potassium: 10 mg, Cholesterol: 0 mg

CREAMY AVOCADO SPREAD

PREPARATION TIME: 5 min
COOKING TIME: None
MODE OF COOKING: No Cooking
SERVINGS: 4 (2 Tbsp per serving)
INGREDIENTS:

- 1 ripe avocado
- 1 Tbsp lime juice
- 1 Tbsp extra-virgin olive oil
- 1/2 tsp garlic-infused olive oil
- 1/4 tsp salt
- 1/4 tsp ground cumin

DIRECTIONS:

1. In a small bowl, mash the avocado until smooth.

2. Stir in lime juice, extra-virgin olive oil, garlic-infused olive oil, salt, and cumin.
3. Mix until well combined and creamy. Serve as a spread on toast, sandwiches, or as a dip for vegetables.

TIPS:

- For a bit of heat, add a pinch of red pepper flakes.
- Use immediately to prevent browning, or store with a piece of plastic wrap pressed against the surface.

N.V.: Calories: 100, Fat: 9g, Carbs: 5g, Protein: 1g, Sugar: 0g, Sodium: 150 mg, Potassium: 250 mg, Cholesterol: 0 mg

ZESTY LEMON TAHINI SAUCE

PREPARATION TIME: 5 min
COOKING TIME: None
MODE OF COOKING: No Cooking
SERVINGS: 6 (2 Tbsp per serving)
INGREDIENTS:

- 1/4 cup tahini
- 2 Tbsp lemon juice
- 1 Tbsp water (or more for thinning)
- 1/2 tsp ground cumin
- 1/4 tsp salt
- 1/4 tsp paprika

DIRECTIONS:

1. In a small bowl, whisk together tahini, lemon juice, water, ground cumin, salt, and paprika until smooth.
2. Adjust the consistency with more water if necessary.
3. Serve over grilled vegetables, as a dip, or drizzle over grain bowls.

TIPS:

- Add a clove of roasted garlic for extra flavor.
- This sauce thickens as it sits; stir in additional water before serving if needed.

N.V.: Calories: 80, Fat: 7g, Carbs: 3g, Protein: 2g, Sugar: 0g, Sodium: 130 mg, Potassium: 60 mg, Cholesterol: 0 mg

ROASTED RED PEPPER SAUCE

PREPARATION TIME: 10 min
COOKING TIME: 15 min
MODE OF COOKING: Blending
SERVINGS: 6 (2 Tbsp per serving)
INGREDIENTS:

- 2 large red bell peppers, roasted and peeled
- 1/4 cup extra-virgin olive oil
- 1 Tbsp red wine vinegar
- 1 tsp smoked paprika
- 1/2 tsp salt
- 1/4 tsp black pepper

DIRECTIONS:

1. Roast the red bell peppers on a grill or directly over a gas flame until charred on all sides.
2. Place the roasted peppers in a bowl and cover with plastic wrap to steam for 10 minutes.
3. Peel the skins off the peppers and remove the seeds.
4. In a blender, combine the roasted peppers, olive oil, red wine vinegar, smoked paprika, salt, and black pepper.
5. Blend until smooth and creamy. Adjust seasoning to taste.

TIPS:

- Use as a pasta sauce, sandwich spread, or dip for bread.
- Store in an airtight container in the refrigerator for up to 5 days.

N.V.: Calories: 70, Fat: 7g, Carbs: 3g, Protein: 1g, Sugar: 1g, Sodium: 170 mg, Potassium: 100 mg, Cholesterol: 0 mg

FRESH HERB PESTO

PREPARATION TIME: 10 min
COOKING TIME: None
MODE OF COOKING: No Cooking
SERVINGS: 6 (2 Tbsp per serving)
INGREDIENTS:

- 1 cup fresh basil leaves
- 1/4 cup fresh parsley leaves
- 1/4 cup pine nuts or walnuts
- 1/4 cup extra-virgin olive oil
- 2 Tbsp nutritional yeast (optional for cheesy flavor)
- 1 Tbsp lemon juice
- 1/4 tsp salt
- 1/4 tsp black pepper

DIRECTIONS:

1. In a food processor, pulse the basil, parsley, and pine nuts until finely chopped.
2. Add the lemon juice, nutritional yeast (if using), salt, and black pepper.
3. With the processor running, slowly drizzle in the olive oil until the mixture is smooth and well combined.
4. Adjust seasoning to taste and serve over pasta, grilled meats, or as a spread.

TIPS:

- For a thicker pesto, reduce the amount of olive oil.
- Store in a sealed jar in the refrigerator for up to a week, or freeze in ice cube trays for later use.

N.V.: Calories: 90, Fat: 9g, Carbs: 2g, Protein: 1g, Sugar: 0g, Sodium: 120 mg, Potassium: 80 mg, Cholesterol: 0 mg

SPICY MUSTARD SAUCE

PREPARATION TIME: 5 min
COOKING TIME: None
MODE OF COOKING: No Cooking
SERVINGS: 8 (1 Tbsp per serving)
INGREDIENTS:

- 1/4 cup Dijon mustard
- 1/4 cup whole-grain mustard
- 2 Tbsp apple cider vinegar
- 1 Tbsp maple syrup
- 1/2 tsp smoked paprika
- 1/4 tsp cayenne pepper (optional for extra heat)

DIRECTIONS:

1. In a small bowl, whisk together Dijon mustard, whole-grain mustard, apple cider vinegar, maple syrup, smoked

paprika, and cayenne pepper (if using).

2. Adjust seasoning to taste and serve as a dip, spread, or marinade.

TIPS:

- This sauce pairs well with grilled meats, roasted vegetables, or as a sandwich spread.
- Store in an airtight container in the refrigerator for up to 2 weeks.

N.V.: Calories: 15, Fat: 0g, Carbs: 3g, Protein: 0g, Sugar: 1g, Sodium: 150 mg, Potassium: 20 mg, Cholesterol: 0 mg

LEMON HERB BUTTER SAUCE

PREPARATION TIME: 5 min
COOKING TIME: 5 min
MODE OF COOKING: Stovetop
SERVINGS: 4
INGREDIENTS:

- 1/4 cup lactose-free butter
- 2 Tbsp lemon juice
- 1 tsp lemon zest
- 1 Tbsp fresh parsley, chopped
- 1 Tbsp fresh chives, chopped
- Salt and pepper to taste

DIRECTIONS:

1. In a small saucepan, melt the lactose-free butter over medium heat.
2. Stir in lemon juice, lemon zest, and fresh herbs.
3. Season with salt and pepper to taste.
4. Cook for 1-2 minutes, stirring occasionally, until the sauce is well combined and fragrant.
5. Remove from heat and serve immediately over grilled fish, chicken, or vegetables.

TIPS:

- For added flavor, add a pinch of garlic-infused olive oil.
- This sauce pairs beautifully with seafood and steamed vegetables.

N.V.: Calories: 90, Fat: 9g, Carbs: 1g, Protein: 0g, Sugar: 0g, Sodium: 60 mg, Potassium: 15 mg, Cholesterol: 20 mg

CREAMY DILL SAUCE

PREPARATION TIME: 5 min
COOKING TIME: None
MODE OF COOKING: No Cooking
SERVINGS: 6 (2 Tbsp per serving)
INGREDIENTS:

- 1/2 cup lactose-free Greek yogurt
- 1 Tbsp lemon juice
- 1 Tbsp fresh dill, chopped
- 1 tsp Dijon mustard
- 1/4 tsp salt
- 1/4 tsp black pepper

DIRECTIONS:

1. In a small bowl, whisk together lactose-free Greek yogurt, lemon juice, fresh dill, Dijon mustard, salt, and black pepper until smooth.
2. Adjust seasoning to taste.
3. Serve immediately or refrigerate until ready to use. This sauce pairs well with salmon, chicken, or roasted vegetables.

TIPS:

- Store in an airtight container in the refrigerator for up to 3 days.
- Add a clove of roasted garlic for an extra depth of flavor.

N.V.: Calories: 25, Fat: 1g, Carbs: 2g, Protein: 2g, Sugar: 1g, Sodium: 90 mg, Potassium: 60 mg, Cholesterol: 2 mg

SPICY TOMATO BASIL SAUCE

PREPARATION TIME: 5 min
COOKING TIME: 20 min
MODE OF COOKING: Stovetop
SERVINGS: 4
INGREDIENTS:

- 1 Tbsp garlic-infused olive oil
- 1 can (14.5 oz) diced tomatoes
- 1/4 cup fresh basil, chopped
- 1/2 tsp red pepper flakes
- 1 tsp balsamic vinegar
- Salt and pepper to taste

DIRECTIONS:

1. In a medium saucepan, heat garlic-infused olive oil over medium heat.
2. Add the diced tomatoes, red pepper flakes, and balsamic vinegar. Stir well.
3. Bring the mixture to a simmer and cook for 15-20 minutes, stirring occasionally, until the sauce thickens.
4. Stir in fresh basil and season with salt and pepper to taste.
5. Serve over pasta, grilled chicken, or as a dipping sauce.

TIPS:

- For a smoother sauce, blend it with an immersion blender before adding the basil.
- Store leftovers in the refrigerator for up to 5 days.

N.V.: Calories: 60, Fat: 2g, Carbs: 10g, Protein: 2g, Sugar: 6g, Sodium: 220 mg, Potassium: 350 mg, Cholesterol: 0 mg

COCONUT CURRY SAUCE

PREPARATION TIME: 5 min
COOKING TIME: 10 min
MODE OF COOKING: Stovetop
SERVINGS: 4
INGREDIENTS:

- 1 cup coconut milk (full fat)
- 1 Tbsp red curry paste
- 1 Tbsp fresh ginger, grated
- 1 Tbsp lime juice
- 1 tsp coconut sugar
- 1/4 tsp salt

DIRECTIONS:

1. In a medium saucepan, combine coconut milk, red curry paste, grated ginger, lime juice, coconut sugar, and salt.
2. Bring to a simmer over medium heat, stirring until the curry paste is fully dissolved.
3. Cook for 5-10 minutes, allowing the flavors to meld and the sauce to thicken slightly.

4. Serve over rice, noodles, or grilled vegetables.

TIPS:

- Add a splash of fish sauce or soy sauce for extra umami.
- Garnish with fresh cilantro and lime wedges for added freshness.

N.V.: Calories: 120, Fat: 12g, Carbs: 4g, Protein: 1g, Sugar: 2g, Sodium: 220 mg, Potassium: 200 mg, Cholesterol: 0 mg

TANGY MANGO SAUCE

PREPARATION TIME: 10 min
COOKING TIME: None
MODE OF COOKING: Blending
SERVINGS: 4
INGREDIENTS:

- 1 ripe mango, peeled and diced
- 2 Tbsp lime juice
- 1 Tbsp maple syrup
- 1 tsp fresh ginger, grated
- 1/4 tsp salt

DIRECTIONS:

1. In a blender, combine diced mango, lime juice, maple syrup, grated ginger, and salt.
2. Blend until smooth and creamy.
3. Serve as a dipping sauce for grilled chicken, fish, or spring rolls.

TIPS:

- For a spicy kick, add a pinch of red pepper flakes.
- Store in an airtight container in the refrigerator for up to 3 days.

N.V.: Calories: 40, Fat: 0g, Carbs: 11g, Protein: 0g, Sugar: 9g, Sodium: 60 mg, Potassium: 120 mg, Cholesterol: 0 mg

GARLIC-INFUSED OLIVE OIL SAUCE

PREPARATION TIME: 5 min
COOKING TIME: 5 min
MODE OF COOKING: Stovetop
SERVINGS: 4
INGREDIENTS:

- 1/4 cup garlic-infused olive oil
- 1 tsp lemon juice

- 1 tsp fresh parsley, chopped
- 1/4 tsp red pepper flakes
- Salt and pepper to taste

DIRECTIONS:
1. In a small saucepan, heat the garlic-infused olive oil over low heat.
2. Stir in lemon juice, fresh parsley, red pepper flakes, salt, and pepper.
3. Cook for 1-2 minutes until fragrant.
4. Remove from heat and serve over pasta, roasted vegetables, or as a dipping sauce for bread.

TIPS:
- For a milder flavor, reduce the amount of red pepper flakes.
- Store in a sealed jar in the refrigerator for up to a week.

N.V.: Calories: 80, Fat: 9g, Carbs: 0g, Protein: 0g, Sugar: 0g, Sodium: 60 mg, Potassium: 10 mg, Cholesterol: 0 mg

MEDITERRANEAN HERB BLEND

PREPARATION TIME: 5 min
COOKING TIME: None
MODE OF COOKING: No Cooking
SERVINGS: 8 (2 tsp per serving)
INGREDIENTS:
- 2 Tbsp dried oregano
- 2 Tbsp dried basil
- 1 Tbsp dried thyme
- 1 Tbsp dried rosemary, crushed
- 1 tsp dried parsley
- 1 tsp garlic-infused olive oil (optional)

DIRECTIONS:
1. In a small bowl, combine dried oregano, basil, thyme, rosemary, and parsley.
2. Stir in garlic-infused olive oil if using for added flavor.
3. Store in an airtight container and use as a seasoning for meats, roasted vegetables, or in marinades.

TIPS:
- This blend is great for sprinkling on grilled chicken or fish before cooking.
- Mix with olive oil to create a quick herb-infused oil for dipping bread.

N.V.: Calories: 5, Fat: 0g, Carbs: 1g, Protein: 0g, Sugar: 0g, Sodium: 0 mg, Potassium: 10 mg, Cholesterol: 0 mg

SMOKY BBQ RUB

PREPARATION TIME: 5 min
COOKING TIME: None
MODE OF COOKING: No Cooking
SERVINGS: 8 (2 tsp per serving)
INGREDIENTS:
- 1 Tbsp smoked paprika
- 1 Tbsp brown sugar or coconut sugar
- 1 tsp ground cumin
- 1 tsp ground mustard
- 1 tsp garlic powder
- 1/2 tsp ground black pepper
- 1/2 tsp salt
- 1/4 tsp cayenne pepper (optional for heat)

DIRECTIONS:
1. In a small bowl, mix together smoked paprika, brown sugar, cumin, mustard, garlic powder, black pepper, salt, and cayenne pepper (if using).
2. Store in an airtight container and rub onto meats or vegetables before grilling or roasting.

TIPS:
- This rub is perfect for ribs, chicken, or even roasted sweet potatoes.
- For a wet marinade, mix the rub with a bit of olive oil and lemon juice.

N.V.: Calories: 10, Fat: 0g, Carbs: 2g, Protein: 0g, Sugar: 1g, Sodium: 120 mg, Potassium: 30 mg, Cholesterol: 0 mg

INDIAN CURRY SPICE BLEND

PREPARATION TIME: 5 min
COOKING TIME: None
MODE OF COOKING: No Cooking
SERVINGS: 8 (2 tsp per serving)
INGREDIENTS:
- 2 Tbsp ground turmeric
- 1 Tbsp ground coriander

- 1 Tbsp ground cumin
- 1 tsp ground ginger
- 1 tsp ground cinnamon
- 1/2 tsp ground cardamom
- 1/2 tsp cayenne pepper (optional for heat)

DIRECTIONS:

1. In a small bowl, combine ground turmeric, coriander, cumin, ginger, cinnamon, cardamom, and cayenne pepper.
2. Mix well and store in an airtight container.
3. Use to season curries, rice dishes, or roasted vegetables.

TIPS:

- For a quick curry, sauté onions, garlic, and your choice of protein, then add this spice blend and coconut milk.
- Add a pinch of this blend to soups for an instant flavor boost.

N.V.: Calories: 10, Fat: 0g, Carbs: 2g, Protein: 0g, Sugar: 0g, Sodium: 5 mg, Potassium: 50 mg, Cholesterol: 0 mg

MEXICAN TACO SEASONING

PREPARATION TIME: 5 min
COOKING TIME: None
MODE OF COOKING: No Cooking
SERVINGS: 8 (2 tsp per serving)
INGREDIENTS:

- 1 Tbsp chili powder
- 1 Tbsp ground cumin
- 1 tsp paprika
- 1 tsp garlic powder
- 1 tsp onion powder
- 1/2 tsp dried oregano
- 1/2 tsp salt
- 1/4 tsp black pepper

DIRECTIONS:

1. In a small bowl, mix together chili powder, ground cumin, paprika, garlic powder, onion powder, oregano, salt, and black pepper.

2. Store in an airtight container and use to season ground meat, beans, or vegetables for tacos.

TIPS:

- Add 1/4 cup of water to the seasoning and meat or beans while cooking for a saucy taco filling.
- This blend can also be used as a seasoning for grilled chicken or shrimp.

N.V.: Calories: 10, Fat: 0g, Carbs: 2g, Protein: 0g, Sugar: 0g, Sodium: 120 mg, Potassium: 30 mg, Cholesterol: 0 mg

ITALIAN SEASONING BLEND

PREPARATION TIME: 5 min
COOKING TIME: None
MODE OF COOKING: No Cooking
SERVINGS: 8 (2 tsp per serving)
INGREDIENTS:

- 1 Tbsp dried basil
- 1 Tbsp dried oregano
- 1 Tbsp dried thyme
- 1 tsp dried rosemary, crushed
- 1 tsp dried marjoram
- 1/2 tsp garlic powder
- 1/2 tsp onion powder

DIRECTIONS:

1. In a small bowl, combine dried basil, oregano, thyme, rosemary, marjoram, garlic powder, and onion powder.
2. Mix well and store in an airtight container.
3. Use to season pasta sauces, pizza, or roasted vegetables.

TIPS:

- Mix with olive oil and vinegar for a quick salad dressing.
- Add a pinch to scrambled eggs or omelets for an Italian twist.

N.V.: Calories: 5, Fat: 0g, Carbs: 1g, Protein: 0g, Sugar: 0g, Sodium: 2 mg, Potassium: 10 mg, Cholesterol: 0 mg

CAJUN SPICE BLEND

PREPARATION TIME: 5 min
COOKING TIME: None
MODE OF COOKING: No Cooking
SERVINGS: 8 (2 tsp per serving)
INGREDIENTS:

- 1 Tbsp paprika
- 1 Tbsp garlic powder
- 1 Tbsp onion powder
- 1 tsp dried thyme
- 1 tsp dried oregano
- 1/2 tsp cayenne pepper
- 1/2 tsp black pepper
- 1/2 tsp salt

DIRECTIONS:

1. In a small bowl, mix together paprika, garlic powder, onion powder, thyme, oregano, cayenne pepper, black pepper, and salt.
2. Store in an airtight container and use to season meats, fish, or vegetables.

TIPS:

- Use this blend to season shrimp or chicken before grilling or sautéing.
- Add to rice or quinoa for a flavorful side dish.

N.V.: Calories: 10, Fat: 0g, Carbs: 2g, Protein: 0g, Sugar: 0g, Sodium: 120 mg, Potassium: 30 mg, Cholesterol: 0 mg

Measurement Conversion Table

Volume Measurements

US Measurement	Metric Measurement
1 tsp (tsp)	5 milliliters (ml)
1 tbsp (tbsp)	15 milliliters (ml)
1 fluid ounce (fl oz)	30 milliliters (ml)
1 Cup	240 milliliters (ml)
1 pint (2 Cs)	470 milliliters (ml)
1 quart (4 Cs)	0.95 liters (L)
1 gallon (16 Cs)	3.8 liters (L)

Weight Measurements

US Measurement	Metric Measurement
1 ounce (oz)	28 grams (g)
1 pound (lb)	450 grams (g)
1 pound (lb)	0.45 kilograms (kg)

Length Measurements

US Measurement	Metric Measurement
1 inch (in)	2.54 centimeters (cm)
1 foot (ft)	30.48 centimeters (cm)
1 foot (ft)	0.3048 meters (m)
1 yard (yd)	0.9144 meters (m)

Temperature Conversions

Fahrenheit (°F)	Celsius (°C)
32°F	0°C
212°F	100°C
Formula: (°F - 32) x 0.5556 = °C	Formula: (°C x 1.8) + 32 = °F

Oven Temperature Conversions

US Oven Term	Fahrenheit (°F)	Celsius (°C)
Very Slow	250°F	120°C
Slow	300-325°F	150-165°C
Moderate	350-375°F	175-190°C
Moderately Hot	400°F	200°C
Hot	425-450°F	220-230°C
Very Hot	475-500°F	245-260°C

CHAPTER 12: CONCLUSION AND FINAL THOUGHTS

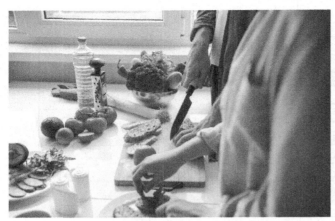

As we wrap up this culinary journey through the practical and flavorful world of low-FODMAP dining, it's a good moment to reflect on how far we've come together. Making significant changes to our diet, especially for health reasons, can feel daunting at first. Yet, with each recipe and each improved meal, we gain more than just new cooking skills; we craft a lifestyle that champions our health and enriches our everyday life.

When I first embarked on creating the "Quick & Easy Low-FODMAP Diet Cookbook," my aim was to convert the complex maze of dietary guidelines into a simple, joyous path forward for you. It has been about breaking down the myths, understanding the why's and how's, and, most importantly, ensuring that you never feel restricted or bored by your meal options. This cookbook was designed not only as a guide but as a companion in your kitchen (and journey to better health), helping you to navigate the low-FODMAP diet with confidence and creativity.

What delights me most is imagining you, the reader, flipping through these pages, perhaps marking a recipe to try or smiling over a newfound favorite that didn't upset your stomach but instead brought comfort and joy. These pages hold not just recipes but stepping stones towards a more comfortable and enjoyable life, free from the distress and discomfort that digestive woes can bring.

As you continue to implement the principles and recipes you've discovered, remember that every individual's body is unique. The key is to tailor these suggestions to meet your specific needs and responses, making adjustments as your body advises. Stay connected with your healthcare provider, and let them guide you based on the feedback your body provides.

In final thoughts, embarking on a low-FODMAP diet is less about facing restrictions and more about discovering a new spectrum of culinary possibilities. It's about transforming challenges into opportunities for creativity, learning, and health a journey well worth embarking on. Here's to many more delicious, gut-friendly meals ahead, to health, happiness, and a life filled with culinary discovery!

12.1 OVERVIEW OF THE LOW-FODMAP JOURNEY

Embarking on the low-FODMAP journey is akin to exploring a new landscape. It's a path that many tread with a blend of hope and hesitation, due in part to past struggles with digestive health that have perhaps led to frustration and discomfort. Yet, as with any journey, the start is about preparing: understanding the map, packing the right supplies, and setting out with a spirit of adventure.

The low-FODMAP diet isn't just a list of foods to avoid; it's a discovery process that involves learning how specific types of carbohydrates affect your body. These carbohydrates, found in a surprisingly wide range of foods, can ferment in the gut and cause the all-too-familiar symptoms of IBS and other digestive challenges. The journey begins by breaking down which carbohydrates to minimize and understanding the benefits this could hold for your long-term wellbeing.

Phase One: **Elimination** For many, the journey kicks off with the elimination phase. This stage is about putting aside high-FODMAP foods to give your body a rest from their fermenting effects. Imagine this phase as an experiment, a way to cleanse the palate to better understand the nuances of your body's true reaction to various foods. It's an essential step, yet one often met with resistance or fear of missing out. This fear feeds the misconception that such a diet will be dull or excessively restrictive. However, flipping the script to see this as a period of culinary exploration in seasoning, texture, and cooking methods opens up a world of enjoyment and creativity.

Phase Two: **Reintroduction** As essential as the elimination phase is, it's equally important not to view it as permanent. The next leg of the journey involves reintroducing different FODMAP groups back into your diet, one at a time. This methodical, careful process allows you to pinpoint exactly which foods trigger symptoms. It's a phase of acute learning and self-discovery, requiring patience and precision. Here, many find it helpful to keep a food diary, noting down what they eat and how it affects their body, fostering a deeper connection and understanding of their digestive health.

Phase Three: **Personalization** Finally, the most rewarding part of the journey: personalization. This stage is when the low-FODMAP diet transcends from a regimen to a lifestyle. Based on the information gathered in the reintroduction phase, you can craft a diet that fits perfectly with your body's unique needs, balancing nourishment and pleasure without discomfort. This final phase is about building a diet that you love, that also loves you back, allowing you to live freely without the constant worry of digestive upset.

Throughout these phases, one thing becomes exceedingly clear: this is not just about avoiding discomfort but about embracing a fuller, more vibrant way of eating and living. It shifts from what you can't eat to focusing on what you can the rich flavors, the fresh ingredients, and the joy of cooking meals that feel good to eat.

Our passages through each phase are as varied as the landscapes we inhabit. For some, the journey may be swift and relatively straightforward, yielding clear results that are easy to interpret. For others, it may involve more complex patterns of sensitivity, requiring extended periods of tweaking and adjustment.

There are common experiences, though, that many share on this diet. Discovering hidden triggers in favorite foods can be disheartening, but it also empowers you to make informed choices. The culinary creativity that blooms from restriction can be another unexpected delight, pushing you to try new ingredients or cooking techniques you might never have considered otherwise. There's also a significant emotional component the relief from finally understanding what has been causing discomfort can be incredibly liberating.

Moreover, there's the aspect of community and support. Engaging with others who are on a similar path can offer comfort and insight. Sharing experiences and recipes, venting about setbacks, and celebrating successes together build a collective strength that reinforces personal commitment.

Yet, just as critical as community, is the guidance and monitoring by health professionals. Regularly consulting with a healthcare provider ensures that your low-FODMAP journey is not only effective but also safe. This collaboration is crucial for adapting the diet to meet other nutritional needs or health conditions, ensuring that you remain well-nourished and vibrant.

In closing, the low-FODMAP diet is more than just a temporary change. It is both a science and an art the science of understanding the biochemical impacts of what we eat on our bodies, and the art of crafting delightful, satisfying meals within this framework. Over time, it teaches resilience and adaptability valuable life skills that extend far beyond the kitchen.

Embarking on this journey may seem formidable at first, but with each small step, it can lead to profound changes in not only digestive health but overall quality of life. With the right tools, knowledge, and spirit of exploration, adapting to a low-FODMAP lifestyle can be a fulfilling, revelatory, and deeply nourishing experience.

12.2 SUSTAINING A LOW-FODMAP LIFESTYLE

Moving from the initial stages of adjusting to a low-FODMAP diet to fully embracing it as a sustainable lifestyle is akin to cultivating a garden. It's about nurturing and maintaining the growth you've begun, monitoring the environment, and making adjustments as necessary so that the garden of your health continues to thrive season after season.

Sustaining a low-FODMAP lifestyle requires a blend of knowledge, adjustment, and most importantly, resilience. It's not merely about adhering to dietary rules but integrating this knowledge into a personalized eating plan that fits seamlessly into your day-to-day life, enhancing your quality of life without feeling burdensome.

Long-Term Management

In the long term, managing a low-FODMAP diet is about creating balance. It's about moving from strict avoidance to a more nuanced understanding of how various foods affect you personally. Once you have identified your triggers in the reintroduction phase, you can incorporate a wider variety of foods while keeping those triggers in check. This doesn't mean living in perpetual restriction; rather, it's recalibrating your diet so that you can enjoy a broad spectrum of foods without discomfort.

Regular Re-evaluation

The body changes, and so too can its responses to different foods. Regularly reassessing your FODMAP tolerance is crucial. This might mean conducting another elimination and reintroduction phase annually or as symptoms change or return. This isn't a step backward but rather a proactive approach to stay aligned with your body's current state and needs.

Educating Yourself and Others

Staying informed is key to sustaining any health-related lifestyle. As research around FODMAPs grows, new findings might adjust what we understand about these compounds and their effects. Keeping up with this research, possibly with the help of a healthcare provider or a dietitian specializing in FODMAPs, will ensure you are always operating with the most current information. Moreover, educating those around you family, friends, colleagues about your dietary needs can make social dining and gatherings far less stressful. When your close circle understands the reasons behind your food choices, they can become supportive participants in your health journey, making accommodations when needed or even exploring low-FODMAP recipes themselves.

Integration into Daily Living

For sustainability, integrating the low-FODMAP diet into your daily routine is essential. This might mean finding quick, simple meal prep strategies that keep you on track even during busy weeks or incorporating mindfulness practices to better understand your body's signals and responses to different foods. Meal planning can play a significant role here, helping to avoid last-minute decisions that might not be in line with your dietary needs.

Support Systems

Having a support system, whether online or in person, can greatly enhance your ability to maintain a low-FODMAP lifestyle. Community groups, whether local or online, can offer advice, empathy, and shared experiences. These networks can be invaluable, not just for the support but for the exchange of practical tips like great low-FODMAP products, recipes, or coping strategies for travel and holidays.

Psychological Considerations

The psychological impact of managing a chronic digestive condition should not be underestimated. Stress, anxiety, and even depression can accompany conditions like IBS, potentially exacerbating symptoms. Addressing these mental health aspects, whether through therapy, stress-relief practices, or other methods, is crucial. This holistic approach can reinforce your efforts in managing your dietary needs by helping to alleviate mental and emotional triggers of digestive symptoms.

Enjoyment and Experimentation

Finally, cultivating a sense of culinary curiosity and enjoyment is perhaps one of the most sustaining aspects of a low-FODMAP lifestyle. Instead of viewing it as restrictive, embracing the creativity it can inspire in your cooking and eating habits can transform your experience. Exploring new cuisines that naturally complement a low-FODMAP diet, experimenting with alternative ingredients, and celebrating the meals that you can enjoy without discomfort can all contribute to a more positive, sustainable approach.

In essence, sustaining a low-FODMAP lifestyle is about more than just careful eating; it's a vibrant, proactive approach to living well. It involves continuous learning and adaptation, a supportive community, mindful practices, and above all, a commitment to nurturing your well-being through every meal and every choice. With these strategies in place, not only can you manage your digestive

health effectively, but you can also enjoy a rich, full, and flavorful life.

12.3 MOTIVATION FOR ONGOING SUCCESS

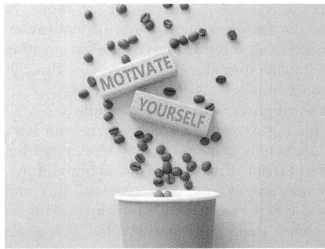

Maintaining motivation on a journey as intricate and personal as the low-FODMAP diet can be akin to navigating a river with its ebb and flow. There are times when the waters are calm and the going is easy, and times when you must paddle harder against the current. The journey to ongoing success with your dietary management is no different it requires perseverance, a positive outlook, and strategies to keep your spirits high and your goals in clear sight.

Rediscovering Your 'Why'

At the start of any endeavor, motivation is often at its peak. This initial surge is powered by the desire for relief and better health. Reminding yourself of why you started can be a powerful motivator to keep going. These reasons might be as straightforward as wanting to enjoy a family meal without discomfort, or as significant as managing symptoms that have overshadowed your life for years. Holding these reasons close can reignite your motivation during times of struggle or monotony.

Celebrating Small Victories

Success in a low-FODMAP lifestyle doesn't only come in the form of big, noticeable changes; it also shows in the subtle shifts in your health and mood. Maybe you've gone a full week without a flare-up, or you've mastered making a delicious low-FODMAP meal that feels gourmet. Celebrating these small victories can provide a sense of accomplishment and a burst of motivation. Each small success builds on the last, creating a momentum that can carry you through tougher days.

Connecting with Success Stories

Hearing or reading about others who have successfully managed their symptoms with a low-FODMAP diet can be incredibly uplifting. These stories can offer practical tips and emotional resonance, providing both a roadmap and the assurance that your goals are attainable. They serve as living proof that the challenges are surmountable and that the rewards of sticking with the diet can be transformative.

Setting Realistic Goals

While it's important to aim high, setting goals that are too ambitious can lead to feelings of failure that sap your motivation. Instead, setting achievable, realistic goals ensures you can meet them and celebrate, fostering positivity and encouraging further progress. These goals can be as simple as incorporating one new low-FODMAP recipe into your meal plan each week or gradually extending the variety of foods in your diet.

Adapting to Your Progress

As you evolve in your low-FODMAP journey, your dietary needs and responses might change, which can affect your motivation. Regularly assessing and adjusting your approach can help keep the diet relevant and effective, renewing your motivation. Sometimes, a small adjustment in your diet or preparation style can reignite your enthusiasm for cooking and eating within this lifestyle.

Keeping It Interesting

Monotony can be a significant demotivator. Keeping the diet interesting by experimenting with global cuisines that are low-FODMAP friendly, or trying new cooking techniques, can inject fun and variety into your meals. This not only keeps your palate excited but also engages your creativity and passion for food, which can be a significant motivational boost.

Building a Support Network

Just as plants thrive best with the support of a trellis, sometimes, you too will need support to grow. Whether it's finding companionship in online communities, joining local support groups, or simply sharing your journey with friends and family, having a support network can provide emotional sustenance. This network can offer not just sympathy but also accountability, which can be critical in keeping you motivated.

Integrating Mindfulness and Positivity

Practicing mindfulness can transform the dietary management from a chore into a more thoughtful practice that ties eating to wellness. By being present in the moment, whether it's savoring your food or listening to your body's reactions post-meal, you connect the act of eating with its impact on your body. This connection can deepen your commitment to the diet and enhance your motivation by constantly relating actions to outcomes.

Reflecting on Your Journey

Taking time to reflect on how far you've come since beginning the low-FODMAP diet can provide a significant motivational boost. Consider keeping a journal or diary from the start of your diet. Looking back over your entries can reveal just how many hurdles you've overcome, reinforcing the benefits of your efforts and renewing your energy for the challenges ahead.

In summary, sustaining motivation in a low-FODMAP lifestyle means finding joy in the journey itself, celebrating every small victory, and continuously adapting to meet your evolving dietary needs. With each day, reminder, and meal, you reaffirm your commitment to a healthier, more vibrant life, fueled by the understanding that the best motivation often comes from within, supported by the community and practices around you.

CHAPTER 13: IN-DEPTH 60-DAY MEAL PLAN

Embarking on a new dietary journey can be both exciting and daunting. As we near the conclusion of our guide, I have tailored a 60-day meal plan that will illuminate your path to a low-FODMAP lifestyle. This chapter isn't simply a set of instructions; it's your own nutritional diary, a companion in the kitchen that whispers secrets to transform your health without sacrificing the joy of eating.

Imagine this: every morning, you wake up already knowing what delightful, gut-friendly meal awaits you. There's no fretting over labels or second-guessing if a meal will trigger discomfort. Over the next two months, you'll savor the simplicity of pre-planned meals ranging from vibrant breakfast bowls to sumptuous dinners, ensuring variety on your plate and consistency in your digestive health. Let's consider the narrative behind this meal plan. It weaves the practicality of low-FODMAP ingredients into your daily meals with an artistry that makes each dish not only a remedy for your body but also a feast for your eyes and palette. You'll find recipes packed with flavors that ensure your food is anything but bland, debunking the myth that dietary food must forsake flavor.

Each week is crafted to gradually integrate more diverse ingredients, building up your confidence in identifying and cooking low-FODMAP meals that please the palate and nurture the gut. As you flip through these pages, I hope you'll feel a growing sense of empowerment and optimism; a testament that a thoughtful approach to eating doesn't just manage symptoms but also enhances the quality of life.

Remember, this meal plan is a starting point. Throughout these 60 days, as your understanding deepens, and your body responds, feel free to tweak and experiment. Adapt recipes to suit your tastes and seasonal availability of produce. This plan is designed to make your journey enjoyable and your transition smooth. Here's to new beginnings and a healthier, happier you!

	breakfast	snack	lunch	snack	dinner
Day 1	Strawberry Yogurt Parfait	Sweet Potato Crostini with Avocado and Pomegranate	Caprese Salad with Quinoa	Decadent Chocolate Avocado Mousse	Sweet Potato and Black Bean Tacos
Day 2	Cozy Vanilla Chai Latte Oatmeal	Zucchini Chips	Tofu Scramble with Spinach and Tomatoes	Spicy Roasted Chickpeas	One-Pot Beef and Cabbage Stir-Fry
Day 3	Warm Banana and Cinnamon Quinoa	Cucumber and Hummus Bites	Mediterranean Veggie Pita Sandwich	Caprese Skewers with Balsamic Glaze	Low-FODMAP Chicken and Spinach Frittata
Day 4	Scrambled Eggs with Spinach and Feta	Greek Yogurt with Berries and Almonds	Grilled Chicken Avocado Wrap	Cucumber Canapés with Smoked Salmon	Herb-Roasted Chicken with Lemon and Rosemary
Day 5	Vanilla Soufflé	Baked Polenta Bites with Tomato and Basil	Tempeh Fajitas with Peppers and Onions	Crispy Kale Chips	Low-FODMAP Chicken Alfredo
Day 6	Veggie-Packed Omelet	Roasted Carrot and Zucchini Sticks	Warm Quinoa and Roasted Vegetable Salad	Chocolate Coconut Macaroons	Grilled Eggplant and Zucchini Stack with Tomato and Basil
Day 7	Sweet Potato and Avocado Breakfast Bowl	Grilled Pineapple with Lime and Mint	Turkey and Swiss Lettuce Wraps	Vegan Avocado Toast with Radishes and Sesame Seeds	One-Pot Italian Sausage and Rice Skillet
Day 8	Berry Quinoa Breakfast Bowl	Smoked Salmon Cucumber Bites	Avocado Toast with Poached Egg	Lemon Poppy Seed Muffins	Easy Turkey Meatloaf
Day 9	Baked Pumpkin Oatmeal	Stuffed Cucumber Bites	Quinoa and Kale Salad with Lemon Vinaigrette	Prosciutto-Wrapped Asparagus	Shrimp and Vegetable Skewers
Day 10	Avocado & Spinach Breakfast Smoothie	Quick Guacamole with Tortilla Chips	Simple Tomato and Cucumber Salad	Baked Sweet Potato Fries	Roasted Vegetable and Lentil Salad

	breakfast	snack	lunch	snack	dinner
Day 11	Strawberry and Almond Butter Oatmeal Bowl	Blueberry Lemon Parfait	Shrimp and Avocado Salad	Shrimp Cocktail with Lemon-Herb Dip	One-Pot Lemon Garlic Chicken with Quinoa
Day 12	Quick Quinoa Breakfast Bowl	Quick Avocado Toast with Tomato	Zucchini and Lemon Soup	Vegan Zucchini Fritters	Zucchini Noodles with Pesto and Cherry Tomatoes
Day 13	Savory Oatmeal with Spinach and Egg	Quick Veggie Wrap	Tempeh Stir-Fry with Vegetables	Decadent Chocolate Avocado Mousse	Low-FODMAP Turkey Meatballs with Marinara Sauce
Day 14	Tropical Quinoa Breakfast Bowl	Polenta Bites with Roasted Red Pepper	Crispy Baked Tofu with Lemon and Herbs	Stuffed Mini Bell Peppers with Herbed Goat Cheese	Quick and Easy Beef Stir-Fry
Day 15	Simple Oatmeal with Strawberries	Grilled Banana Boats	Avocado and Citrus Salad	Vegan Guacamole and Veggie Sticks	Grilled Vegetable Skewers with Quinoa
Day 16	Warm Cinnamon Quinoa Porridge	Greek Yogurt with Berries and Almonds	Grilled Veggie and Hummus Wrap	Baked Zucchini Fries with Parmesan	One-Pot Ground Beef and Potato Hash
Day 17	Hearty Pumpkin Spice Pancakes	Baked Peaches with Cinnamon Almond Crumble	Tuna Salad Collard Wraps	Raspberry Coconut Macaroons	Low-FODMAP Chicken and Vegetable Stir-Fry
Day 18	Creamy Polenta with Sautéed Spinach and Egg	Baked Polenta Bites with Tomato and Basil	Quick Tuna Salad with Cucumber	Chocolate-Dipped Strawberries	One-Pot Shrimp and Vegetable Pasta
Day 19	Banana Oat Pancakes	Blueberry Lemon Parfait	Tempeh Tacos with Avocado	Vegan Zucchini Fritters	One-Pot Chicken and Vegetable Curry
Day 20	Lemon Ricotta Pancakes	Stuffed Cucumber Bites	Spinach and Strawberry Salad with Lemon Vinaigrette	Chocolate Coconut Macaroons	Low-FODMAP Beef Stroganoff

	breakfast	snack	lunch	snack	dinner
Day 21	Berry Quinoa Breakfast Bowl	Tropical Fruit Salad with Lime Dressing	Chicken and Avocado Wrap	Caprese Skewers with Balsamic Glaze	Roasted Vegetable and Lentil Salad
Day 22	Creamy Coconut Rice Pudding	Smoked Salmon Cucumber Bites	Spicy Chicken Salad Wrap	Crispy Kale Chips	Baked Salmon with Dill and Citrus
Day 23	Almond Flour Lemon Cookies	Quick Guacamole with Tortilla Chips	Maple-Soy Glazed Tofu	Shrimp Cocktail with Lemon-Herb Dip	One-Pot Chicken and Rice
Day 24	Strawberry and Almond Butter Oatmeal Bowl	Grilled Pineapple with Lime and Mint	Veggie-Packed Hummus Wrap	Peanut Butter Chocolate Chip Cookies	Low-FODMAP Macaroni and Cheese
Day 25	Hearty Pumpkin Spice Pancakes	Quick Avocado Toast with Tomato	Warm Quinoa and Roasted Vegetable Salad	Spicy Roasted Chickpeas	Grilled Vegetable Skewers with Quinoa
Day 26	Quick Quinoa Breakfast Bowl	Sweet Potato Crostini with Avocado and Pomegranate	Grilled Chicken Avocado Wrap	Baked Zucchini Fries with Parmesan	One-Pot Beef and Cabbage Stir-Fry
Day 27	Cozy Vanilla Chai Latte Oatmeal	Roasted Carrot and Zucchini Sticks	Zucchini and Lemon Soup	Cucumber Canapés with Smoked Salmon	Low-FODMAP Chicken and Spinach Frittata
Day 28	Sweet Potato and Avocado Breakfast Bowl	Grilled Peaches with Balsamic Glaze	Tuna Salad Collard Wraps	Vegan Guacamole and Veggie Sticks	Low-FODMAP Chicken Alfredo
Day 29	Fluffy Coconut Rice Pudding	Cucumber and Hummus Bites	Tempeh Tacos with Avocado	Chocolate-Dipped Strawberries	Roasted Vegetable and Quinoa Bowl
Day 30	Warm Cinnamon Quinoa Porridge	Zucchini Chips	Shrimp and Avocado Salad	Raspberry Coconut Macaroons	Low-FODMAP Beef Stroganoff
	breakfast	snack	lunch	snack	dinner
Day 31	Fluffy Coconut Pancakes	Polenta Bites with Roasted Red Pepper	Mediterranean Veggie Pita Sandwich	Prosciutto-Wrapped Asparagus	One-Pot Ground Beef and Potato Hash
Day 32	Veggie-Packed Omelet	Baked Polenta Bites with Tomato and Basil	Caprese Salad with Quinoa	Vegan Avocado Toast with Radishes and Sesame Seeds	One-Pot Italian Sausage and Rice Skillet
Day 33	Scrambled Eggs with Spinach and Feta	Grilled Pineapple with Lime and Mint	Tempeh Fajitas with Peppers and Onions	Baked Sweet Potato Fries	Low-FODMAP Turkey Meatballs with Marinara Sauce
Day 34	Warm Banana and Cinnamon Quinoa	Roasted Carrot and Zucchini Sticks	Avocado Toast with Poached Egg	Decadent Chocolate Avocado Mousse	Shrimp and Vegetable Skewers
Day 35	Avocado & Spinach Breakfast Smoothie	Sweet Potato Crostini with Avocado and Pomegranate	Simple Tomato and Cucumber Salad	Stuffed Mini Bell Peppers with Herbed Goat Cheese	One-Pot Lemon Garlic Chicken with Quinoa
Day 36	Baked Pumpkin Oatmeal	Smoked Salmon Cucumber Bites	Spinach and Strawberry Salad with Lemon Vinaigrette	Lemon Poppy Seed Muffins	Quick and Easy Beef Stir-Fry
Day 37	Simple Oatmeal with Strawberries	Zucchini Chips	Turkey and Swiss Lettuce Wraps	Raspberry Coconut Macaroons	Sweet Potato and Black Bean Tacos
Day 38	Tropical Quinoa Breakfast Bowl	Quick Veggie Wrap	Quinoa and Kale Salad with Lemon Vinaigrette	Peanut Butter Chocolate Chip Cookies	One-Pot Chicken and Vegetable Curry
Day 39	Savory Oatmeal with Spinach and Egg	Baked Peaches with Cinnamon Almond Crumble	Tempeh Stir-Fry with Vegetables	Vegan Guacamole and Veggie Sticks	One-Pot Shrimp and Vegetable Pasta
Day 40	Banana Oat Pancakes	Cucumber and Hummus Bites	Grilled Veggie and Hummus Wrap	Vegan Zucchini Fritters	Herb-Roasted Chicken with Lemon and Rosemary

	breakfast	snack	lunch	snack	dinner
Day 41	Lemon Ricotta Pancakes	Grilled Peaches with Balsamic Glaze	Crispy Baked Tofu with Lemon and Herbs	Chocolate-Dipped Strawberries	Zucchini Noodles with Pesto and Cherry Tomatoes
Day 42	Strawberry Yogurt Parfait	Grilled Banana Boats	Avocado and Citrus Salad	Crispy Kale Chips	Low-FODMAP Chicken and Vegetable Stir-Fry
Day 43	Creamy Polenta with Sautéed Spinach and Egg	Stuffed Cucumber Bites	Quick Tuna Salad with Cucumber	Cucumber Canapés with Smoked Salmon	Grilled Eggplant and Zucchini Stack with Tomato and Basil
Day 44	Cozy Vanilla Chai Latte Oatmeal	Tropical Fruit Salad with Lime Dressing	Tofu Scramble with Spinach and Tomatoes	Spicy Roasted Chickpeas	Easy Turkey Meatloaf
Day 45	Scrambled Eggs with Spinach and Feta	Quick Guacamole with Tortilla Chips	Spicy Chicken Salad Wrap	Caprese Skewers with Balsamic Glaze	One-Pot Chicken and Vegetable Curry
Day 46	Warm Cinnamon Quinoa Porridge	Smoked Salmon Cucumber Bites	Mediterranean Veggie Pita Sandwich	Shrimp Cocktail with Lemon-Herb Dip	Roasted Vegetable and Quinoa Bowl
Day 47	Avocado & Spinach Breakfast Smoothie	Quick Avocado Toast with Tomato	Tuna Salad Collard Wraps	Vegan Avocado Toast with Radishes and Sesame Seeds	Low-FODMAP Beef Stroganoff
Day 48	Fluffy Coconut Rice Pudding	Grilled Peaches with Balsamic Glaze	Simple Tomato and Cucumber Salad	Chocolate Coconut Macaroons	One-Pot Shrimp and Vegetable Pasta
Day 49	Sweet Potato and Avocado Breakfast Bowl	Blueberry Lemon Parfait	Maple-Soy Glazed Tofu	Baked Zucchini Fries with Parmesan	Quick and Easy Beef Stir-Fry
Day 50	Quick Quinoa Breakfast Bowl	Polenta Bites with Roasted Red Pepper	Avocado Toast with Poached Egg	Prosciutto-Wrapped Asparagus	One-Pot Ground Beef and Potato Hash
	breakfast	snack	lunch	snack	dinner
Day 51	Banana Oat Pancakes	Tropical Fruit Salad with Lime Dressing	Zucchini and Lemon Soup	Spicy Roasted Chickpeas	Sweet Potato and Black Bean Tacos
Day 52	Veggie-Packed Omelet	Zucchini Chips	Tempeh Tacos with Avocado	Caprese Skewers with Balsamic Glaze	One-Pot Lemon Garlic Chicken with Quinoa
Day 53	Vanilla Soufflé	Quick Veggie Wrap	Caprese Salad with Quinoa	Vegan Zucchini Fritters	Low-FODMAP Turkey Meatballs with Marinara Sauce
Day 54	Baked Pumpkin Oatmeal	Baked Polenta Bites with Tomato and Basil	Warm Quinoa and Roasted Vegetable Salad	Shrimp Cocktail with Lemon-Herb Dip	Shrimp and Vegetable Skewers
Day 55	Tropical Quinoa Breakfast Bowl	Quick Guacamole with Tortilla Chips	Chicken and Avocado Wrap	Cucumber Canapés with Smoked Salmon	Low-FODMAP Macaroni and Cheese
Day 56	Fluffy Coconut Pancakes	Sweet Potato Crostini with Avocado and Pomegranate	Veggie-Packed Hummus Wrap	Lemon Poppy Seed Muffins	Low-FODMAP Chicken Alfredo
Day 57	Hearty Pumpkin Spice Pancakes	Grilled Banana Boats	Shrimp and Avocado Salad	Stuffed Mini Bell Peppers with Herbed Goat Cheese	One-Pot Italian Sausage and Rice Skillet
Day 58	Warm Banana and Cinnamon Quinoa	Baked Peaches with Cinnamon Almond Crumble	Grilled Chicken Avocado Wrap	Peanut Butter Chocolate Chip Cookies	Grilled Vegetable Skewers with Quinoa
Day 59	Creamy Coconut Rice Pudding	Greek Yogurt with Berries and Almonds	Spinach and Strawberry Salad with Lemon Vinaigrette	Chocolate-Dipped Strawberries	One-Pot Chicken and Rice
Day 60	Almond Flour Lemon Cookies	Roasted Carrot and Zucchini Sticks	Tempeh Fajitas with Peppers and Onions	Baked Sweet Potato Fries	Baked Salmon with Dill and Citrus

CHAPTER 14: USEFUL APPENDICES

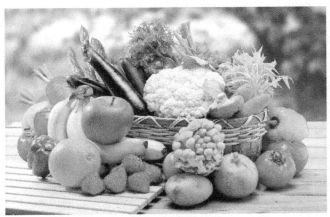

Navigating a Low-FODMAP diet can sometimes feel like deciphering a complex map without a guide. You've gathered your tools: flavorful recipes, meal plans, and insights on how each dish could suit your dietary needs. But what about those moments of uncertainty or the need for quick references as you stand in the grocery aisle? That's what this chapter is here for, to serve as your personal compass in those often-overwhelming scenarios.

In the day-to-day reality of managing a restrictive diet, especially one as nuanced as the Low-FODMAP, questions bound to arise or situations that need a quick fix are inevitable. Perhaps you've stood puzzled in front of myriad food labels, trying to remember if a specific additive is a friend or foe to your gut. Or maybe you're planning a dinner and need to quickly check which spices align with both sensational taste and dietary safety. That's where these appendices shine, providing clear, easy-access information to support your journey without the hassle.

Here, we lay down a comprehensive shopping guide designed to transform your grocery shopping from a stressful task into an enjoyable adventure. It demystifies labels for you, pointing out what to look for and what to avoid, ensuring every product in your cart is a safe choice.

Additionally, keeping a food journal becomes less of a chore and more of an insightful activity with our specially designed template, tailored to spot patterns and identify what works best for your body. And for those pressing queries that catch you off guard, a section dedicated to FAQs ensures you're never left searching for answers for too long.

This chapter is created with the purpose to make your Low-FODMAP pathway as clear and straightforward as possible, equipped with tools that not only provide immediate solutions but also deepen your understanding and comfort with this diet. Whether it's a quick lookup or a detailed consultation of the lists and guides, consider this as your trusty sidekick in the culinary adventures of sensitive digestion. Let it enhance your confidence and expand the horizons of what a Low-FODMAP diet can be a harmonious blend of health management and culinary delight.

14.1 COMPREHENSIVE SHOPPING GUIDE

Imagine you're embarking on a treasure hunt, not in search of gold, but for gut-friendly nourishment that keeps your days both active and free from discomfort. Mastering the art of shopping on a Low-FODMAP diet doesn't require a magnifying glass or a detective's hat; rather, it calls for knowledge, awareness, and a trusty guide this comprehensive shopping guide.

Navigating the supermarket aisles can be daunting. Bright packages and bold claims vie for your attention, yet here you are, searching for labels that signify safety and comfort for your sensitive digestive system. Begin your journey by embracing the perimeter of the grocery store. This is where fresh produce, meats, and dairy products typically lie. These staples generally make a safer bet on a Low-FODMAP diet, provided you adhere to the right choices and portions.

Fresh Fruits and Vegetables: A Colorful Array of Options Start with the produce section. Low-FODMAP fruits like oranges, strawberries, and grapes offer that burst of sweetness without the subsequent pain. In greens, bell peppers, carrots, and tomatoes (fresh, not canned) are colorful partners in your culinary creations. The key here is moderation; even Low-FODMAP foods can tip the scales if consumed in large amounts.

However, steer clear of garlic and onions, notorious disruptors for FODMAP-sensitive stomachs. But this doesn't mean meals must lack flavor. Chives, green onion tops, and an array of herbs and spices can enhance dishes, letting you savor the flavors without the fear.

Choose Proteins that Propel Your Day Venturing further in, the protein section beckons. Lean meats like chicken, turkey, and certain cuts of beef are excellent building blocks for a Low-FODMAP meal. If you're eyeing seafood, most fresh fish are compliant, but always double-check for added sauces or marinades that might sneak in high-FODMAP ingredients. Eggs, too, are great heroes in this journey, versatile and safe.

For plant-based dieters, tofu and tempeh make great choices, but avoid high-FODMAP beans and lentils unless very well-cooked and still, in small servings. You will find that these protein sources can be combined in numerous ways through your weekly meals without repetition.

Navigating the Dairy Dilemma In the dairy aisle, the waters might seem murky. Lactose is a major FODMAP offender. Thankfully, lactose-free milk and yogurts are often easy to find and clearly labeled. Almond milk or coconut milk are your allies here, but watch for additives. Traditional cheeses like cheddar, Swiss, and parmesan are typically lower in lactose and can be enjoyed without much worry.

Grains that Ground You In the realm of breads and cereals, choose grains wisely. Look for gluten-free options not because gluten is a FODMAP issue, but because wheat, barley, and rye products also contain high levels of fructans. Fortunately, quinoa, rice, and oatmeal are filling and safe alternatives that serve as excellent bases for a variety of meals.

Snacks: Your Safe Havens For many, snacks are the trickiest part, as most convenient options are laden with high-FODMAP enemies. Search for snacks labeled gluten-free often a good indicator they're free of wheat, barley, and rye. Rice cakes, certain nuts like walnuts and peanuts, and even a homemade trail mix can be lifesavers between meals. Just remember to balance quantity with caution to maintain a harmonious gut.

The Inner Isles: Tread with Care Sauces, soups, and condiments require a keen eye. Many of these can hide high-FODMAP ingredients like onion or garlic powder. As a safe practice, equip yourself with knowledge of alternative products that are specifically marketed as Low-FODMAP. These products are crafted to exclude gut-aggravating ingredients and can be great staples in your pantry.

Remember, too, that reading labels is a skill that grows sharper with practice. Terms like 'inulin', 'HFCS' (high-fructose corn syrup), and any syrups or chicory roots are signals to put the product back on the shelf. Embrace brands that cater to FODMAP-sensitive shoppers, as they often disclose all ingredients transparently, understanding the necessity for such clarity in conditions like yours.

Lastly, as you approach the checkout counter, with your cart filled with your safe and delicious choices, remember the importance of planning. Fewer impulsive buys lead to better health outcomes. Crafting a versatile yet structured weekly meal plan one that both excites and nurtures will convert your shopping trip from a puzzle to a pleasure.

Armed with this guide, grocery shopping transforms into an empowering adventure, charting a course through a world flourished with suitable, savory selections. Each item in your cart isn't just food; it's a building block to a healthier, more vibrant you, leading to a life not dictated by dietary restrictions but enriched by the possibilities within them.

14.2 FODMAP FOOD JOURNAL

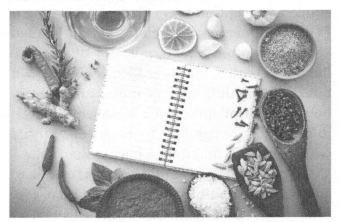

Embarking on the Low-FODMAP journey is akin to becoming a detective in your own kitchen and dining adventures, sleuthing out what agrees with your body and what sets off a less-than-pleasant reaction. This detective work, however, is not complete without its most crucial tool: a food journal. Maintaining a FODMAP food journal can transform an often-frustrating trial-and-error process into an insightful and manageable exploration of what nourishments truly suit you.

Imagine sitting down to a meal, hopeful and hungry. You've made choices that seem safe, but the response might still be unpredictable. Here's where your food journal becomes invaluable. Not merely a log of meals, but a personal database that captures your dietary habits, symptoms, and the ultimate effects of specific foods. It allows you to document and correlate the inputs and outcomes, offering insights that are as nourishing to your understanding as the food is to your body.

Creating Your Food Journal: The Setup
Starting a food journal doesn't require elaborate tools a simple notebook, a digital app, or a dedicated diary all serve the purpose.

The key is consistency and detail. Each entry serves as a snapshot of your day's dietary intake.

Begin by recording every meal, snack, and drink consumed. Note the quantities too, as they might impact how you react even to low-FODMAP foods. Additionally, consider the context of your meals. Foods that you tolerate well on one day may not sit well when you're stressed, lacking sleep, or pairing them with different foods.

Adding Layers of Detail: Symptoms and Mood Post-meal reflections are just as crucial. Note any symptoms that arise be they digestive troubles, headaches, or fatigue and the time they occur. This immediacy helps in establishing closer connections between your meals and their effects. Mood and stress levels before and after meals also offer insights, as emotional states can significantly impact digestive processes. Over time, patterns will likely emerge, painting a clearer picture of which foods trigger symptoms and under what circumstances.

Beyond Food and Symptoms: Environmental and Lifestyle Factors The weather, your location during meals, the interval between eating and sleeping all these factors can influence digestion. By including these nuances in your journal, you create a comprehensive overview of your health interplay. Did a quick lunch on a busy workday result in discomfort? Have leisurely weekend meals at home left you feeling better? These observations are pivotal in fine-tuning your diet.

Reflect, Review, and Revise: Using Your Journal for Long-Term Insights Periodically, it's beneficial to sit down with your journal and review the accumulated entries. Search for trends and try to understand the why behind the reactions. Perhaps certain spices, although Low-FODMAP, consistently show up in entries marked by discomfort. Or maybe dairy alternatives you believed to be safe are frequently coinciding with symptoms.

Armed with months of detailed notes, you'll approach your dietitian's office not as a patient lost in confusion but as an informed partner in your health journey. This review process isn't just about omitting troublesome foods but about celebrating and increasing the intake of those that consistently nourish and satisfy you without repercussions.

Empowerment Through Patterns and Triggers Over time, this journal will evolve into a testament of your proactive journey towards digestive health. It empowers you with knowledge and control over your symptoms, shifting the perspective of the Low-FODMAP diet from restrictive to liberating. Patterns from your journal will guide alterations to your diet, tailored precisely to your body's needs, ensuring that your nutrient intake is optimized without comfort compromise.

As days turn into weeks, and weeks into months, your food journal will become richer with data and insights. It evolves, just as your understanding of your body's responses evolves. And with each entry, you're not just filling out pages you're sketching a map that leads to better health, greater understanding, and ultimately, a happier life.

Concluding Thoughts: Your Dynamic, Digestive Diary Think of your food journal not simply as a record but as a dialogue with your body a continuous conversation that grows deeper and more insightful with each meal. Just as no two people are alike, no journal will look the same; it's a personal mosaic composed of dietary details, physical reactions, emotional states, and environmental contexts, all interacting in unique ways.

In this journey, your food journal is both your compass and companion, helping navigate through the complexities of dietary management to a destination of digestive peace and personal empowerment. Through diligent logging, thoughtful reviewing, and strategic revising, this simple tool paves the way to a more predictable and enjoyable eating experience, providing a blend of scientific observation and personal reflection that is uniquely yours.

14.3 COMMON QUESTIONS AND SOLUTIONS

Embarking on a Low-FODMAP diet introduces a spectrum of common queries and concerns. Every journey is studded with questions, some as frequent as meal times themselves. You're not alone in wondering about the practicalities of managing such a specific diet, especially when balancing it with a dynamic lifestyle. Here, we'll delve into those recurring questions and provide solutions that harmonize knowledge with everyday practicality.

How do I handle dining out? Navigating restaurant menus while following a Low-FODMAP diet can seem daunting. Start by reviewing menus online before visiting to plan what you can eat. Don't hesitate to call ahead and discuss your dietary needs; many chefs are willing to accommodate. Choose dishes with simple, whole ingredients and ask for dressings or sauces on the side. Opt for grilled or roasted entrees and clarify that your food should be prepared without garlic or onions.

What about social situations and family gatherings? Social events need not be a source of stress. When attending a gathering, bring a dish that you know is safe for you to eat. This not only ensures you'll have something suitable to enjoy, but it also provides an opportunity to share with others how delicious Low-FODMAP foods can be. Be open with hosts about your dietary restrictions it's about your health, after all.

Is there a simple way to explain the diet to friends and family? Explaining the Low-

FODMAP diet can sometimes feel complex due to its nuances. Describe it as a method to identify foods that trigger digestive symptoms like bloating, gas, and stomach pain. You might mention that it involves eliminating certain common irritants from the diet, which are found in everyday items like wheat, onions, and milk. Emphasize that everyone's triggers are different, which is why personalized insights gained from following the diet are invaluable.

How quickly can I expect to see improvements in my symptoms? Improvements can vary widely among individuals. Some experience relief within the first week, while others may take longer to notice changes. It's important to adhere strictly to the diet during the initial phase and consult with a healthcare provider to track progress and ensure nutritional balance is maintained.

What should I do if I accidentally eat a high-FODMAP food? Mistakes happen, and it's important not to be too hard on yourself. If you consume a high-FODMAP food, take note of it in your food journal and observe how your body responds. This information can be valuable for your understanding of personal thresholds. Support your body by returning to known safe foods and consider natural digestion aids like peppermint tea.

Can I ever reintroduce high-FODMAP foods into my diet? Yes, the goal of the Low-FODMAP diet is not permanent elimination but rather identification of your personal triggers. The reintroduction phase is a structured process where one high-FODMAP food is carefully reintroduced at a time while monitoring symptoms. This stage helps define what quantities and combinations of these foods are tolerable, aiming for the broadest possible diet without triggering symptoms.

How do I manage the Low-FODMAP diet on a tight budget? Eating fresh, whole foods while avoiding many processed items is a cornerstone of the Low-FODMAP diet, which can sometimes be costly. However, strategies like buying seasonal produce, choosing generic brands, and cooking large meals to freeze for later can help manage costs. Prioritize low-FODMAP pantry staples like rice, eggs, and frozen vegetables that can stretch meals further.

What supplements should I consider while on this diet? Before starting any supplements, consult with a healthcare professional to discuss your specific needs. Typically, depending on your dietary restrictions and what your normal diet lacks, you might consider fiber supplements if you find it difficult to obtain adequate fiber from Low-FODMAP vegetables and fruits. Similarly, calcium and vitamin D might be needed if dairy is significantly limited.

How do I maintain a balanced diet while following a restrictive plan? It's essential to ensure diversity within the bounds of Low-FODMAP options. Incorporate a variety of allowed fruits, vegetables, proteins, and whole grains to maintain nutrient intake. Regularly consult with a nutritionist to ensure your diet remains balanced and provides all necessary nutrients. Each question you have as you navigate this diet contours the path to a lifestyle harmonized with your health needs. Remember, this diet is a learning process, where each observation about how foods affect you is a stepping stone to a better quality of life. While challenges arise, each solution drawn from insights enhances the ease of living with dietary restrictions, proving that a proactive attitude and the right knowledge can significantly alleviate the hurdles encountered on this journey. Embrace each day with curiosity and a readiness to adapt, using these solutions as guideposts along the way.

Made in the USA
Las Vegas, NV
19 December 2024